Pregnancy Guide for Men

A Month-By-Month Handbook for First-Time Dads to Support Your Partner and Enjoy Your Baby

Peter Neel

© Copyright 2023 – Peter Neel – All rights reserved

The content within this book may not be reproduced, duplicated, or transmitted without direct written permission from the author or publisher.

Under no circumstances will any blame or legal responsibility be held against the publisher, or author, for any damages, reparation, or monetary loss due to the information contained within this book, either directly or indirectly.

Legal Notice

This book is copyright protected. It is for personal use only. You cannot amend, distribute, sell, use, quote, or paraphrase any part, or the content within this book, without the author's or publisher's consent.

Disclaimer Notice

Please note that the information contained within this document is for educational and entertainment purposes only. All effort has been executed to present accurate, up-to-date, and reliable, complete information. No warranties of any kind are declared or implied. Readers acknowledge that the author does not render legal, financial, medical, or professional advice.

Table of Contents

Introduction 5
Chapter 1: Embracing the Journey of Becoming a Father 8
    The Miraculous Process of Conception 8
    Getting Ready for an Emotional Roller Coaster 10
    Preparing for the First Doctor's Appointment 12
    Celebrating the Exciting News of "We Are Pregnant!" 14
Chapter 2: Entering the First Month 17
    Recognizing Your Vital Role as a Father 17
    Revealing the Early Indicators of Pregnancy 19
    Supporting Her During the Early Stages of Pregnancy 21
    Empowering the Journey With Empathy 23
Chapter 3: Harmonizing the Second Month of Pregnancy 26
    Getting a Grip on Early Pregnancy Changes 26
    Fostering Bonds Through Effective Communication 28
    Creating a Healthy Pregnancy Diet Plan 30
    Making Your Home Environment Healthier and Safer 32
Chapter 4: Listening to the Song of the Third Month 35
    Seeing the First Ultrasound Photo of the Baby 35
    Admiring the Growing Pregnancy Bump 37
    Extending Support Amid the Risk of Miscarriage 39
    Promoting Gentle Exercises for Fitness 41
Chapter 5: Navigating the Emotions of the Fourth Month 44
    Coping With Hormonal Changes During Mid-Pregnancy 44
    Nurturing Patience Amid the Turbulence 46
    Boosting Her Confidence and Self-Esteem 48
    Dealing With Pregnancy-Related Sexual Issues 50
Chapter 6: Embarking on the Fifth Month's Journey 53
    Embracing the Excitement and Apprehension of the Gender Reveal 53
    The Importance and Benefits of Antenatal Classes for Parenting 55
    Strategizing for a Financially Secure Future 57
    Fostering a Bond With the Baby Through the Power of Touch 59

Cultivating a Supportive Community of Prepared Fathers 62

Chapter 7: Unveiling the Peaceful Oasis of the Sixth Month................ 64

Alleviating Her Pregnancy Discomfort With Massage Therapy 64

Creating a Tranquil Nursery for Your Little One 66

Finding Common Ground on Parenting Strategies..68

Getting Emotionally Ready for the Arrival of the New Life..................................71

Chapter 8: Crafting the Seventh Month's Symphony 74

Connecting With the Unborn Baby Through Your Voice......................................74

Baby Showers – A Time to Celebrate Your Unborn Child 76

Preparing Yourself for the Childbirth Experience..78

Prioritizing Mother and Baby's Well-Being With Regular Health Check-Ups ... 80

Chapter 9: Immersing in the Eighth Month's Prelude..........................83

Offering Support Through Late Pregnancy Challenges 83

Making Sure You Are a Part of the Birth Plan..85

Embarking on a D-Day Hospital Tour..87

Preparing With Assembled Baby Gear 89

Chapter 10: Getting Ready for the Ninth Month's Grand Finale 92

True Signs of Labor Versus False Alarms..92

Being Her Pillar of Support Throughout Labor 94

Experiencing the Miraculous Moment of Birth..96

Providing Postpartum Support Following Birth 98

Chapter 11: Celebrating the Grand Debut 101

How to Handle the Baby's First Few Days 101

Sharing the Joy and Challenges That Come With Parenting...............................103

Learning Your Newborn's Secret Language 105

Fostering Unconditional Love Through Baby Bonding 107

Chapter 12: Setting Sail on the Continued Journey of Fatherhood 110

Baby Sleep Schedules – How to Get Through Sleepless Nights 110

Help Her Get Over the Baby Blues 112

Cultivating Your Relationship While Embracing Parenthood............................114

Contemplating the Journey and the Evolution Into Fatherhood 116

Embarking on a Parenthood Journey Together 118

Final Words 120

About the Author.. 122

Introduction

In the first glow of morning light, you felt it. A tiny, rhythmic thump-thump-thump against your palm. It was subtle, almost undetectable, but unmistakably real. It was the first kick from the little being your partner is carrying inside of her. A rush of exhilaration swept through you – a blend of awe, happiness, and a touch of anxiety. The reality of becoming a father has just grown more palpable. Suddenly, you realized how much you did not know about pregnancy and all that it entails.

There is a particular kind of quiet panic that you might be feeling right now. After all, you are about to enter a world that has traditionally been the domain of women – pregnancy. Your partner is probably already armed with a stack of pregnancy books, and she has got friends, her mother, and perhaps a sister or two, giving her advice and sharing their experiences. But where does that leave you, the expectant father? You also have questions, fears, and concerns, but resources addressing your unique perspective can feel sparse.

But what if there was a way to navigate these uncertain waters? A guide, designed specifically for you, the expectant father, that walks you through each stage of pregnancy, helping you understand what is happening with your partner's body, the developing baby, and how you fit into this picture. A resource that enables you to share more fully in the pregnancy journey, feel informed, and be a supportive partner in a meaningful way for both of you.

Imagine knowing exactly how to soothe your partner's morning sickness, or understanding why she is experiencing those mood swings. Picture yourself being able to engage in knowledgeable conversations with the healthcare provider, asking relevant questions that show you are not just an onlooker in this process, but an integral part of it. Envision bonding with your child even before they are born, by understanding the developmental milestones happening right under your fingertips as you touch your partner's belly. This is not just about being a spectator in the pregnancy journey; it is about being an active participant, fostering deeper connections, and transforming apprehension into confidence.

This is not knowledge that was acquired overnight. Instead, it is the culmination of extensive research, consultations with healthcare professionals, and the personal experiences of many fathers who have been on the same journey you are embarking upon. It encapsulates years of knowledge, collated and presented in a friendly and accessible manner. While it may not replace medical advice, it surely fills the gap that most conventional pregnancy books leave when addressing the father's role and experience during pregnancy.

While no two pregnancies are the same and every journey is unique, the insights and guidance in this book offer a framework that can empower you. You can go from being unsure and overwhelmed to becoming a confident partner, equipped with the knowledge to navigate these remarkable nine months. By investing your time in understanding pregnancy from the father's perspective, you are not only contributing to a healthier and happier pregnancy for your partner but also establishing the groundwork for a strong bond with your child.

Picture yourself nine months from now. The labor is underway, and your partner is depending on you to be her pillar of strength. How prepared do you want to be in that situation? The knowledge you gain now will directly influence your confidence and your ability to support her during the birthing process. It will shape your first few moments with your child, a memory that will stay with you for life. The clock is ticking, and every day that you are not preparing is a missed opportunity to deepen your understanding and become the supportive partner and father you aspire to be.

For generations, men have been on the outskirts of the pregnancy experience, often feeling helpless, unprepared, and overwhelmed by the transformation happening in their partner's body. They were tossed into the sea of fatherhood, expected to learn to swim as the waves of change and responsibility crashed over them. The journey was daunting, filled with a scramble for piecemeal information, often incomplete or unrelatable, leaving many new fathers feeling isolated and disoriented.

But you are not alone, and you do not have to feel lost. This guide is here to illuminate your path and equip you with the knowledge you need. It is designed for men like you, standing on the precipice of the incredible journey that is fatherhood, seeking guidance and reassurance. This is your handbook, your reference, and your companion for the nine months ahead and beyond. It is time to step forward confidently, to share in the joys and challenges of pregnancy, and to prepare for the unforgettable moment when you welcome your child into the world.

Chapter 1:
Embracing the Journey of Becoming a Father

The Miraculous Process of Conception

The journey of conception begins with a microscopic act of love and unity, something so minute yet profoundly life-changing. It is a miraculous process that unfolds deep within the body, unseen by the naked eye, and yet, its outcomes can be felt, lived, and cherished for a lifetime.

Men, it is essential to understand that your role in conception is as vital as that of your partner. It is not just the act of fertilization; your emotional support, physical health, and lifestyle habits significantly influence this journey. Hence, it is crucial to comprehend that conception is a joint responsibility, one that involves equal contributions from both partners.

Imagine a race where millions of contenders vie for one grand prize. This is precisely what happens during fertilization. Approximately 250 million sperms commence a challenging journey up through the cervix, into the uterus, and finally, toward the fallopian tubes. However, only the strongest and fastest reaches the ovum. It is nature's finest example of survival of the fittest.

This meeting, a single sperm penetrating a mature ovum, kickstarts a fascinating cascade of biological processes. The fertilized egg, now termed a zygote, begins to divide and grow into a cluster of cells as it moves toward the womb. Within approximately a week, this little bundle of cells finds a cozy spot in the uterus to nestle in, marking the start of pregnancy.

The scientific beauty of conception is that it is meticulously timed, finely tuned, and executed with the utmost precision. Yet, it is much more than a mechanical process. Conception symbolizes the creation of a new life, a unique blend of two individuals' genetic material. It embodies the genesis of a new chapter, a new identity – that of being parents.

Men, it is time to cast away the notion that pregnancy is a woman's domain. You are a part of this journey, right from its inception. The healthier your sperm, the better the chances of conception. This means paying attention to your diet, exercise regimen, and habits like alcohol and tobacco consumption.

Also, it is important to comprehend the emotional implications of this journey. For many couples, conception is not an immediate result of their decision to start a family. It could take several attempts, and sometimes, there may be challenges along the way. It is a period that tests your patience, resilience, and emotional strength. Remember, it is not just about "making a baby," it is about supporting each other in this shared journey.

On a practical note, tracking your partner's menstrual cycle can be an excellent first step in understanding the "fertile window," the best time for conception. Apps and digital tools can help with this, but the key is to approach it as a shared responsibility and not a mechanical chore.

Conception is an incredible voyage that requires your active participation, physically and emotionally. As you prepare to embark on this journey, remember, it is the first step in your transformation into a father. The patience, understanding, and support you exhibit now lay the foundation for the nurturing father you will soon become.

In this grand orchestration of life, you are not a mere spectator, but a conductor, orchestrating your symphony of love, life, and legacy.

Getting Ready for an Emotional Roller Coaster

Ever been on a roller coaster? Picture it. The climb up that first steep slope, the anticipation building in your gut, the excitement mixed with a pinch of fear. That is parenthood. And just like that first drop, the moment you hear the words, "We are pregnant," your heart leaps into your throat. The joy is overwhelming, nearly debilitating. Your brain begins to race, envisioning all those cliché moments of throwing a ball in the yard, teaching them how to ride a bike, and reading bedtime stories. But just as quickly, a twinge of anxiety hits, followed by fear and an unsettling feeling of being unprepared. That is all normal. Every father-to-be goes through this whirlwind of emotions. So how do you handle it?

First, breathe. Yes, this is a monumental change, and yes, it is natural to feel overwhelmed. Remember that these feelings are not unique to you. You are not the first man to become a father, and you certainly will not be the last. Allowing yourself to feel this bundle of emotions is the first step in embracing fatherhood. It is okay to be scared. It is okay to be excited. And yes, it is okay to feel both at the same time.

Now, when anxiety seizes you, making you feel like you are teetering on the edge, remember the image of the roller coaster. Like a roller coaster ride, fatherhood is an experience filled with ups and downs. The highs of fatherhood can be incredibly high – seeing your child for the first time, hearing their first word, and witnessing their first steps. But there will also be lows – sleepless nights, dirty diapers, and incessant crying. Embrace these. The lows are as much a part of the journey as the highs. They are what make the joyous moments shine even brighter.

As you navigate this emotional roller coaster, communication is crucial. Share your feelings with your partner. Remember, they are on this ride with you, perhaps feeling even more intense emotions. Being open about your anxieties and fears can help you both feel less alone in this journey. This is a shared experience, and talking about your feelings can strengthen your bond and prepare you both for the coming months.

To help manage your anxiety, take time each day to practice mindfulness. This could be a moment of silence in the morning, a walk in nature, or writing in a journal. These small moments of self-reflection can help you stay grounded in the present and reduce feelings of overwhelm.

Additionally, lean into education. Fear often comes from the unknown. By learning about pregnancy and fatherhood, you can mitigate some of your anxieties. There are countless resources available – from books to online forums – that can give you insight into what to expect in the coming months.

Finally, remember to celebrate! This is an exciting time in your life. Allow yourself to feel the joy and anticipation. Imagine the future with your child, and let those thoughts fuel your happiness.

You are on the precipice of an incredible journey. With all its ups and downs, fatherhood is a ride like no other. Remember, every emotion you are feeling – whether it is excitement, fear, happiness, or anxiety – is normal. Embrace them, communicate them, and most importantly, prepare to enjoy the ride. It is one you will remember for a lifetime.

Preparing for the First Doctor's Appointment

How many times in your life have you been to a doctor's appointment that was not about you? Unless you have accompanied a loved one during an illness or had a previous journey to parenthood, the odds are not many. In an environment where all the questions, examinations, and paperwork are centered around your partner, it is easy to feel like an outsider. But remember, you are in this together. Your presence matters. So, let us delve into your role and what to expect at the first prenatal doctor's appointment.

As you prepare for the first doctor's appointment, you may feel a swirl of emotions, from excitement to nervousness. You are stepping into a world of medical jargon and procedures, most of which are new and confusing. The ultrasound, the tests, and the health history discussions may feel overwhelming. But do not let these dampen your enthusiasm. Instead, see them as integral parts of the journey toward welcoming your little one.

The initial prenatal visit is usually the most comprehensive. The doctor will confirm the pregnancy, determine the due date, and evaluate the mother-to-be's health. This visit may involve several medical procedures like a pelvic exam, Pap smear, blood tests, urine tests, and potentially the first ultrasound to verify the pregnancy's progress. These tests are crucial for identifying any health issues that need attention, assessing the baby's development, and setting a baseline for future comparisons.

Why are these tests necessary? Each one serves a unique purpose. For instance, the blood and urine tests check for specific markers indicating the baby's and mother's health. They can help identify potential complications, such as gestational diabetes or preeclampsia, early. Understanding this can help you better support your partner by encouraging her through these necessary albeit sometimes uncomfortable procedures.

So, what is your role in all of this? While you will not be on the receiving end of any medical procedures, your role is just as crucial. You are there as the chief support officer. Hold your partner's hand, lend an ear to her concerns, and offer comforting words.

Before the appointment, help your partner prepare any questions for the doctor. Amid the flurry of information at the visit, it can be easy to forget important inquiries. You can be the second set of ears, listening keenly to the doctor's responses, and helping your partner remember crucial information.

Your active participation can also extend to learning about healthy pregnancy habits and risk factors. You can commit to a healthier lifestyle together, like quitting smoking if applicable, and ensuring your home is a safe environment for your growing baby.

After the appointment, have a debriefing session together. Discuss the visit, answer her questions if you can, or help seek answers for those that you cannot. These simple actions can make a big difference, reinforcing the fact that you are in this together.

Indeed, the first prenatal visit is more than just a routine medical appointment. It is the start of a shared journey, a voyage you are undertaking together. Embrace it. Engage actively. Ask questions. Provide comfort. Your involvement sets the tone for your journey into fatherhood, a journey that begins long before your baby arrives.

Remember, you are not just an observer. You are an integral part of this process, a beacon of support for your partner. And most importantly, you are about to become a father. So, let the journey begin, starting with the first prenatal doctor's appointment. In doing so, you are taking your first active steps toward welcoming your child into the world.

Celebrating the Exciting News of "We Are Pregnant!"

Remember the first time you gazed into the eyes of your partner and felt that overwhelming feeling of love? Think of that moment now, magnify that emotion tenfold, and you might come close to understanding the inexplicable joy of announcing your forthcoming parenthood. But here is the catch: Along with this excitement, there is a chance you might be feeling a whirlpool of other emotions – anxiety, fear, and uncertainty, all perfectly normal.

Why does this array of feelings occur? Well, life is about to change in ways you have never imagined. You are stepping into the shoes of a father, a nurturer, and a guide. It is not just about you and your partner anymore; there is a new life in the picture, and sharing this colossal news is as much an emotional milestone as it is a logistical one.

Here is the first bit of advice: When it comes to announcing the news about your baby, timing is everything. While you might be thrilled to broadcast the news immediately, it is wise to discuss this with your partner first. When and whom to tell is a decision that should be made together, as a team.

Once you have decided on the timing, ponder how you would like to share this joyous news. Would you prefer a grand announcement at a family gathering, a quiet and intimate sharing with each loved one, or perhaps a creative reveal on social media? Remember, there is no right or wrong method, and the "how" entirely depends on your comfort level and personal preference.

Now, let us address the elephant in the room: The anxiety associated with the announcement. What if your family has certain expectations? How will your colleagues react? What if they do not share your excitement?

Understand this, every change, especially ones as significant as this, can bring a certain degree of tension. People might have opinions, expectations, and a barrage of advice. But here is the thing – this is your journey, shared with your partner, and no one else's opinions should cast a shadow on your happiness.

You might be worried about your workplace reactions, especially about the need for paternity leave or flexible work hours in the future. It is essential to familiarize yourself with your company's policies on parental leave and your legal rights. When you feel ready and comfortable, speak openly with your supervisor. More often than not, you will find that they are supportive and understanding.

Lastly, ensure to create a support network. Pregnancy, childbirth, and parenting are incredibly joyful, but they can also be demanding. Reach out to friends who are parents, join support groups, or forums where you can share your thoughts, experiences, and even fears.

In conclusion, remember, announcing your journey into fatherhood is a moment of pure joy, a celebration of life. It is a journey you and your partner embark on together, a testament to your shared love and commitment. So, hold hands, take a deep breath, and step onto this new path with excitement and positivity, because you are about to experience one of life's most profound joys – parenthood.

Chapter 2:
Entering the First Month

Recognizing Your Vital Role as a Father

Did you ever imagine that one day you would be flipping through a book, searching for answers about how to be a supportive partner during pregnancy? If you have found yourself here, let us start by acknowledging your dedication. Your role as an expectant father is not to be underestimated; it is both crucial and transformative.

Imagine you are about to set sail on a new voyage. The vessel is the mother-to-be; she is the one physically carrying the new life. But you, dear reader, are the indispensable compass and anchor.

Your role as a father begins long before you hold your child for the first time. It starts from the moment you learn about the pregnancy, and in a myriad of ways, both practical and emotional. You may not realize it, but you are already taking on your new role by seeking knowledge to be the best partner you can be.

From a practical perspective, one of the best ways to be supportive is to be involved. Attend prenatal appointments with your partner, as this is not only a way to show you are invested but also an opportunity to understand the process and ask questions. Be proactive in learning about a healthy lifestyle for pregnancy. This does not mean suddenly becoming an expert, but knowing the basics about diet, exercise, and what changes to expect will go a long way.

Another practical aspect is preparing for the arrival of your child. This could mean setting up the nursery, planning finances, or researching childcare options. These tasks, while seemingly ordinary, are concrete ways to contribute and lessen your partner's load.

On the emotional front, providing support might involve understanding and adapting to changes. There will be hormonal fluctuations that could affect your partner's mood and physical well-being. Take time to educate yourself about these changes, and try to empathize. A reassuring hug, a patient ear, or a simple gesture of understanding can often mean more than words.

Remember that your partner might also be dealing with anxieties about the changes her body is undergoing, worries about the delivery, or concerns about becoming a parent. This is where your role as an emotional anchor becomes invaluable. It is okay if you do not have all the answers; sometimes, providing comfort comes from simply acknowledging these fears and offering reassurance.

Indeed, your role as an expectant father is multifaceted and important. This might feel daunting, but it is also an opportunity. It is a chance to deepen your relationship with your partner, to grow as a person, and to begin forming a bond with your unborn child.

Like an anchor stabilizes a ship, your support during this journey is crucial to help steady your partner amid the waves of change. Like a compass, your guidance and involvement will help navigate the voyage toward parenthood. Keep this in mind as you step into this significant role – and embrace the journey that lies ahead.

Revealing the Early Indicators of Pregnancy

It is the early hours of the morning and you are abruptly awakened by your partner rushing to the bathroom. This scenario could be a repeated performance during the first trimester of pregnancy. You might wonder, "What is happening to her?" or "How can I help?" Let us take a closer look at the common early signs of pregnancy and explore practical ways you can support your partner during this transformative period.

Morning Sickness: Despite the name, this wave of nausea can hit at any time of the day or night. For many pregnant women, the heightened sense of smell exacerbates this symptom. A comforting gesture, such as taking on kitchen duties to keep strong food odors at bay, can provide relief for your partner.

Tender, Swollen Breasts: Hormonal changes might make her breasts unusually sensitive. An understanding nod and a gentle touch, instead of a puzzled look, can go a long way. Perhaps, surprise her with a more comfortable maternity bra, signaling your understanding of her physical changes.

Fatigue: If she is feeling tired more often than usual, it is because of the increased levels of the hormone progesterone. Supporting her by taking up more chores, encouraging rest, and ensuring she maintains a balanced diet rich in proteins and iron can help combat fatigue.

Frequent Urination: As the pregnancy progresses, the volume of blood and other fluids in your partner's body will increase, leading to more frequent trips to the bathroom. This might also disturb her sleep. Assure her that it is normal and consider strategizing sleeping arrangements to minimize disturbances.

Food Aversions and Cravings: She might start disliking certain foods while developing a fondness for others. Remember, these changes are primarily driven by hormonal fluctuations. Helping her maintain a balanced diet, making a midnight ice cream run, or simply providing companionship as she navigates these new preferences can be an excellent support strategy.

Mood Swings: Hormonal changes can also trigger mood swings. During these times, she might need reassurance and understanding more than anything. Remember, this is an emotional roller coaster ride for her too. Encourage open conversation about these experiences, providing a safe and non-judgmental space for her to express her feelings.

Understanding these early signs of pregnancy is essential because it demystifies the process, fostering a greater sense of empathy and connection. It also equips you with knowledge, allowing you to offer practical and meaningful support to your partner during this period.

Pregnancy is a shared journey. Just as your partner is learning to adjust to her changing body and fluctuating hormones, you too are learning – about these changes, about patience, empathy, and support. Every trip you make to the store for an unexpected craving, every gentle massage you offer to soothe aches and pains, and every tender word of reassurance, contribute to making this shared journey a deeply bonding and meaningful experience. Your understanding of these symptoms and proactive support will not only comfort your partner but also help you cultivate a deeper connection with each other and your baby-to-be.

Supporting Her During the Early Stages of Pregnancy

Imagine yourself embarking on an incredible journey where the path is uncharted, and the destination is one of life's most profound miracles. Your partner, the person you love more than anyone in the world, is your travel companion. You are not the one carrying the load, but your job is to be the best co-navigator, stepping up to become the strong, compassionate, and supportive partner she needs.

The first trimester, especially, can be quite a roller coaster ride for women. It is during this time that the dreaded morning sickness kicks in for many. This is more than just feeling a bit queasy; it can be a relentless, all-day discomfort. So, how do you help alleviate it? Start by understanding that every woman's experience is different. What works for one might not work for another. Encourage her to eat small meals frequently, and keep bland snacks like crackers or rice cakes nearby, as they are known to help. Certain smells might trigger nausea, so try to avoid strong odors, especially in the kitchen. And when she is having a rough morning, just being there to rub her back or hold her hand can make a world of difference.

While helping with physical discomfort is vital, contributing to a peaceful environment is equally important. Research shows that stress can exacerbate symptoms of morning sickness, so strive to create a calming atmosphere at home. Take on more household chores to give her time to rest. Indulge in activities that relax her – be it watching her favorite movie, playing soothing music, or simply sitting together in quiet companionship. Make sure she knows that you are there for her, ready to provide comfort and care at a moment's notice.

Pregnancy calls for certain lifestyle adjustments, many of which are not easy to make. It is no longer just about her; there is a tiny life blossoming inside that needs protection. As an expectant father, you can lead by example. If she is giving up alcohol or caffeine, show solidarity and give them up too. Adopt a healthier diet and encourage regular gentle exercise. Remember, you are in this together.

Perhaps she loves sushi, but now she cannot have it because of the risk of bacteria and parasites. Or maybe she is a coffee connoisseur, but now has to limit her intake. Sacrifices are hard. Show empathy and appreciation for the adjustments she is making. Surprise her with pregnancy-safe alternatives. Explore decaf options or find recipes for delightful homemade mocktails. These small gestures can go a long way.

The journey of pregnancy is shared, but the physical experience is hers alone. You will not feel the hormonal changes, the nausea, or the body's transformation. But this does not mean you cannot empathize and help. Let her know it is okay to express her discomfort without feeling guilty. Listen to her, offer comfort, and help find solutions. Understand her needs, both spoken and unspoken.

Remember, pregnancy is not just about enduring hardships; it is a beautiful journey that you are taking together, leading to the precious destination of parenthood. Celebrate the little victories, whether it is finding a food that does not trigger nausea or completing a peaceful, stress-free day. Be her cheerleader, her confidant, her rock. And most importantly, be patient and kind, because this journey, with all its challenges and rewards, is a testament to the strength of your love and the family you are about to become.

Empowering the Journey With Empathy

Picture yourself on an uncharted path in the thick of a dense forest. The sky is painted with hues of crimson and gold as the sun begins to set, making the foliage even denser. Suddenly, you hear a soft rustle. You squint your eyes and peer into the twilight. A small, scared animal emerges, trembling and frightened, feeling lost, uncertain, and overwhelmed. What do you do? Your innate reaction would be to soothe, comfort, and guide it, right? Now, let us draw a parallel here. Pregnancy can often feel like navigating an unfamiliar, thick forest for your partner. It is a time when your empathy – that ability to understand, share, and respond to another's emotions – comes into play.

Being empathetic during this time begins with patience. Remember, just like you would not hurry the little animal in the forest, you cannot rush your partner. Pregnancy is a journey with its unique rhythm, and you must respect this pace. Patience is not just about waiting; it is about the attitude while waiting. Even when things get tough, try to wear a smile and radiate positivity. However, avoid false optimism or rushing her to feel "normal." It is okay to let her know that it is all right to have bad days and good days, and she is doing an incredible job.

Next comes understanding. Pregnancy might result in physical discomfort, emotional turmoil, and cognitive shifts for your partner. It is crucial not to dismiss these as "just pregnancy things." Her experiences and feelings are valid and important. Try to imagine yourself in her shoes and consider how you would feel. It will help you better appreciate what she is going through.

Active listening plays an essential role in understanding her better. Practice active listening by being fully present during conversations. This is not just about hearing her words but interpreting the feelings behind them. Reflective phrases like "It sounds like you are feeling ..." or "What I hear you saying is ..." can be incredibly validating and supportive for her.

Being emotionally present is the pillar on which empathy stands. She needs you to be her sanctuary, her haven. Share her happiness, acknowledge her fears, and make space for her uncertainties. Remember, it is not always about fixing problems, but about standing beside her while she navigates them.

At the end of the day, empathy is not about grand gestures but about simple, everyday actions. It is making her a warm cup of tea, it is holding her hand during a doctor's appointment, and it is validating her emotions without judgment. Empathy builds bridges, deepens your relationship, and, most importantly, makes her feel seen, heard, and loved.

In a world that constantly advises us to "walk a mile in someone's shoes," pregnancy is a journey where you cannot exactly do that. However, you can walk beside her, every step of the way, fueling the journey with empathy. Remember, she is not just carrying your child; she is carrying a new world within her. Being empathetic helps you be a part of that world and makes the journey less daunting for both of you. So, let empathy be your compass as you navigate this journey together.

So, dear reader, are you ready to fuel this journey with empathy? Are you prepared to be patient, understanding, and emotionally present for your partner? Remember, the heart of empathy is love, and there is no better way to step into fatherhood.

Chapter 3:
Harmonizing the Second Month of Pregnancy

Getting a Grip on Early Pregnancy Changes

Have you ever observed the spring season's shift? The way the cold, barren winter gradually gives way to the warmth and colors of spring? The change is not always smooth. There is often a lingering chill, sudden showers, the chaos of life emerging everywhere. But through it all, nature's transformation is nothing short of miraculous.

In much the same way, the second month of pregnancy marks a time of profound transformation for the woman carrying new life within her. A silent metamorphosis is taking place, tucked away from the eyes of the world but undoubtedly felt by her. This period signifies one of the most crucial phases in your journey to parenthood, and your understanding of these changes can make all the difference.

The first noticeable physical changes are often the enlargement and darkening of her breasts, a heightened sense of smell, increased urination, fatigue, and, of course, the infamous morning sickness. These changes are predominantly triggered by the flood of pregnancy hormones – primarily hCG, progesterone, and estrogen.

The hormone human chorionic gonadotropin (hCG) is the main culprit behind nausea and vomiting, often referred to as "morning sickness," though it can strike at any time of day. The rapid increase in progesterone and estrogen can trigger mood swings, from elation to despair in a matter of minutes. Imagine riding the world's most unpredictable roller coaster, and you are getting close to understanding how she might feel.

While these changes may seem daunting, and the emotional tides unnerving, they serve an essential purpose. The same hormones causing discomfort also signal to her body to nourish the growing embryo, transforming the uterus into a nurturing haven. The fatigue and nausea are her body's way of slowing her down, reminding her to take care and conserve energy for the development taking place within.

As an expectant father, you might feel helpless watching her endure these challenges. But remember, understanding is the first step toward providing effective support. Instead of feeling sidelined, equip yourself with knowledge, empathize with her experience, and become her pillar of strength.

When she is dealing with morning sickness, make sure she is eating small, frequent meals, and stays hydrated. Even simple gestures, such as being the one to prepare meals or taking over chores, can provide immense relief.

During mood swings, remind yourself that her emotions are being fueled by hormonal changes. Remain patient and supportive. Give her space when she needs it, and offer a comforting presence when she seeks it. Your understanding will reassure her that she is not alone in this journey, providing profound emotional support that is vital during this phase.

The road ahead is not without its bumps, and the changes she is experiencing can be overwhelming. But always remember, these changes are temporary. The transformation happening is magical, bringing you one step closer to the miraculous arrival of your child. Be patient, be understanding, and let love guide your actions.

Understanding and supporting each other during this period can strengthen your bond, not only as partners but as co-creators in the wondrous journey of life. And trust me, when you hold your baby in your arms for the first time, every challenge weathered will be worth it. You are in this together, every step of the way.

Fostering Bonds Through Effective Communication

Recall the moment you first found out about the pregnancy. You felt a whirlwind of emotions, right? A sense of awe, joy, fear, and perhaps a tinge of uncertainty. If you, as a future father, are feeling such a flood of emotions, can you imagine what the mother of your child is going through? Her body and mind are on a roller coaster of hormonal changes. She is bearing the miracle of a new life, and with it, a cauldron of hopes, dreams, expectations, and, yes, fears. And that is where you, the expectant father, play a crucial role – through open, gentle, and honest communication.

Let us imagine a common scenario. Your partner comes home after a long day, exhausted and irritable due to morning sickness, aches, and a sudden revulsion to the smell of coffee she used to adore. She snaps at you for something trivial. Your first instinct might be to snap back, defend yourself, or withdraw. But this is where empathetic communication comes into play.

Here are some practical tips to foster effective communication with your partner:

Empathize, Do Not Solve: When your partner is venting about her discomforts, it is essential to listen with empathy. Resist the urge to provide solutions or fix things unless she asks for them. Sometimes, she might just need a sounding board to voice her frustrations, fears, and anxieties.

Engage in Active Listening: Nod, maintain eye contact and respond appropriately to show you are engaged in the conversation. It is not about just hearing her words but truly understanding the emotions and sentiments behind them.

Express Your Feelings, Too: Communication is a two-way street. It is equally important to express your own fears, hopes, and expectations. Vulnerability fosters closeness and connection. But remember, it is not a competition of who is having a harder time. You are on this journey together.

Discuss Expectations Openly: Do not leave things to assumption. Talk about your expectations from each other during this journey. What kind of support does she need from you? How do you wish to be involved in the pregnancy journey? Discuss, negotiate, and come to a mutual understanding.

Reassure Regularly: Reassurance is an antidote to many fears and anxieties. Regularly reassure your partner of your love, support, and presence throughout the journey.

Now, let us apply these tips to the scenario. Instead of snapping back, you might say, "I see you are exhausted and irritated. This pregnancy is taking a toll on you, right? I am here for you, sweetheart. Is there anything I can do to make you feel better?" This empathetic response opens the door for a conversation rather than an argument, bridging any potential emotional gap between you two.

Remember, these tips are not a one-size-fits-all solution. All relationships, all people, and all pregnancies are unique. Use these tips as a guideline, and adjust them according to your specific circumstances.

Effective communication is like a glue that holds your relationship together, especially in challenging times like pregnancy. Your willingness to communicate openly and honestly can make your partner feel understood, supported, and loved, strengthening your bond as you both journey toward parenthood. After all, as the great relationship expert H. Norman Wright said, "Communication is to a relationship what breathing is to life." Keep the communication lines open, and watch your relationship thrive.

Creating a Healthy Pregnancy Diet Plan

Did you ever imagine that a tiny human being, smaller than a grain of rice, could govern what your partner eats, or rather, what she cannot stand to eat? Welcome to the peculiar world of pregnancy cravings and aversions. Pregnancy is a grand adventure, and much of it is navigated through the kitchen and the dining table. Food plays a vital role, providing the essential nutrients needed for your baby's growth and your partner's health. And as an expectant father, your role is crucial in helping her maintain a balanced diet.

Pregnancy cravings are no myth; they are as real as the child that is growing inside your partner's womb. You might find yourself making midnight runs to the store to satiate your partner's cravings for pickles, ice cream, or anything in between. Sometimes, it might be a specific dish from a certain restaurant, the very thought of which brings a gleam to her eyes.

On the other hand, food aversions can be equally strong. That delicious lasagna she could not get enough of last month? It might turn her stomach now. These shifts in appetite might seem whimsical, but they are a normal part of pregnancy, often linked to hormonal changes.

Now, let us dive into the nutritional needs during pregnancy. In general, your partner's diet should be rich in proteins, carbohydrates, healthy fats, fiber, vitamins, and minerals. Specific nutrients to focus on include folic acid, iron, calcium, and omega-3 fatty acids, all of which are crucial for your baby's development.

The question now is, how can you, as an expectant father, contribute to a healthy pregnancy diet for your partner? First, it is important to understand that you are not just a bystander in this journey, but an active participant.

You can start by encouraging regular meals and snacks to keep up energy levels and prevent nausea. Keep the pantry stocked with nutrient-rich foods like fruits, vegetables, whole grains, lean proteins, and dairy products. Help your partner stay hydrated by ensuring she always has a bottle of water at hand.

If she is experiencing morning sickness, try to identify any triggers. Often, simple adjustments, like avoiding spicy or fatty foods, or eating smaller meals more frequently, can help alleviate the symptoms.

Another important aspect is to be aware of foods to avoid during pregnancy. Certain foods carry a risk of foodborne illnesses that could harm your partner or the baby. For instance, undercooked or raw seafood, unpasteurized dairy products, and raw or undercooked meat are generally best avoided.

Finally, remember to provide emotional as well as nutritional support. Your partner's body is changing, and she may struggle with issues related to body image and self-esteem. Reassure her that she is beautiful, doing a great job and that both of you are in this together.

The road to parenthood is paved with shared meals, midnight cravings, and morning sickness. But it is also filled with moments of joy, shared laughter, and growing anticipation. And as you navigate this journey together, remember that the best dish you can offer your partner is your unwavering love and support.

Making Your Home Environment Healthier and Safer

Remember that day when you received the good news of your upcoming parenthood? You embarked on a voyage of a lifetime, filled with boundless joy, excitement, and, let us face it, a bit of nervousness too. But now, as reality sets in, it is time for some concrete actions. As you enter the second month, an essential step is to make your home a safe haven for your partner and the baby on the way. The home environment plays a significant role in the health and well-being of your expectant partner.

Perhaps you have never given much thought to the cleaning products stacked in your cupboard. They do a great job of keeping your surfaces sparkling and your clothes smelling fresh, right? But did you know many conventional cleaning products are a cocktail of chemicals that could potentially harm your partner and the baby?

A study from the Royal College of Obstetricians and Gynaecologists in 2013 suggested that pregnant women should avoid food packaging, ready meals, and even new furniture to limit their exposure to chemicals that could harm their babies. The same goes for many cleaning products, which often contain ingredients like phthalates and parabens, both linked to hormonal disruption and potential developmental issues for the fetus. While occasional exposure is unlikely to cause harm, why take a chance when safer alternatives exist?

Here are some practical steps to make your home environment healthier and safer:

Opt for Natural Cleaning Products: Many brands offer "green" or natural cleaning products that are free from harsh chemicals. Look for those certified as safe for both environmental and human health. Do remember, "natural" does not always mean safe, so always check the ingredient list.

DIY Cleaning Solutions: If you are into DIY projects, why not try making your own cleaning solutions? For instance, a mixture of vinegar and water works wonders for windows, while baking soda makes a non-abrasive scrub for sinks and tubs. You will be surprised how easy and cost-effective it can be, and the peace of mind you will get is priceless.

Ventilation is Key: Regularly air out your home, especially after cleaning or painting, to disperse any lingering chemicals in the air. If you have any painting projects planned, ensure to use VOC-free paint. Volatile organic compounds (VOCs) are common in regular paint and can cause headaches and respiratory issues.

Careful With the Garden: If you love your garden and tend to it regularly, remember to choose natural fertilizers and pesticides. Many conventional gardening products contain harmful substances that could be harmful if inhaled or absorbed through the skin.

As the expecting father, your role in this detoxifying process is not just a supportive one, but a proactive one. After all, it is not just about creating a healthy environment for your partner and the baby, but also about paving the way for a healthier lifestyle for your soon-to-be expanded family.

Yes, making changes can feel overwhelming at first. But remember, you are not alone in this. Your partner is in this with you, and together, you are making your home a safe nest for your little one. You are embarking on an exciting journey – one that brings responsibilities but also unmatchable joys. With every change you make, remember, you are one step closer to meeting your little bundle of joy.

Chapter 4:
Listening to the Song of the Third Month

Seeing the First Ultrasound Photo of the Baby

Can you recall the first time you felt truly amazed? That moment when reality surpassed every expectation, every hope, and every dream you had? The day you see your baby on the ultrasound for the first time will be one such moment. An ethereal spectacle, a life-altering experience, a visceral bond formed through the grainy shades of the ultrasound monitor. This chapter is here to guide you through that transcendent moment, brimming with anticipation and joy.

Seeing your baby on the ultrasound monitor for the first time is akin to witnessing a miracle unfold before your eyes. It is as if a veil has been lifted from a hidden world, revealing your tiny creation. This glimpse into the world of your unborn child will take you to a new level of connection. A connection that transcends words and lives in the language of shared heartbeat, wonder, and silent promises of undying love.

But let us take a step back. You are walking into the ultrasound room, a cool, quiet place of low light and palpable expectation. Your heart is thundering, and your palms might be damp with anxiety. Rest assured, that is completely natural. As the ultrasound technician guides you through the process, each beat of your heart is a countdown to the moment that will redefine your life forever.

When the screen flickers to life, you will see a nebulous world of shadows and forms. Amid this cosmos, there is a tiny heartbeat, a flutter in the monochrome stillness – your baby. It might look like a peanut, a tiny blip on the screen, but it is a part of you. It is the physical embodiment of the love between you and your partner.

You might not realize it at that moment, but this first ultrasound is more than just a glimpse of your baby. It is the first page of a lifelong story that you will write together. It is the initiation of a dialogue that will unfold over the years, a dialogue of laughter, tears, hopes, dreams, triumphs, and trials.

So, what should you do to celebrate this monumental moment? Here are a few suggestions. Frame the ultrasound picture and put it in a place where you will see it every day. This could be on your bedside table, at your workspace, or even as a screensaver on your phone. Share this joyous moment with your loved ones, spreading the cheer and involving them in your journey. You could even hold a small gathering or a party to commemorate this special occasion.

Remember, the joy of this experience is not confined to the ultrasound room. It follows you and it transforms you. It turns men into fathers, and couples into families. As you step out of the ultrasound room, you are stepping into a new world, a world where you are no longer just a man, but a father-to-be.

Remember, the anticipation of meeting your little one can bring a rush of emotions, from joy to anxiety. It is important to support each other during this time. Each day of this journey is a shared experience, a memory you are creating together. Embrace it, live it, and love it. This is just the beginning, and what a beautiful beginning it is!

In the end, the most valuable piece of advice one can give you is to be present. Be there in every moment, every heartbeat, and every breath. Because while this journey is nine months in the making, the memories you are creating will last a lifetime. This first ultrasound is not just a doctor's visit, it is a landmark on your journey to fatherhood. Enjoy the journey, treasure the moments, and remember – you are not alone. You have the best companion you could ask for, your partner in this voyage of creation and love.

Admiring the Growing Pregnancy Bump

There is a moment in every pregnancy that changes everything. A point at which the abstract idea of "We are having a baby" transforms into a tangible reality. Often, it is when the baby bump starts to show, a vivid sign of the life burgeoning within. Suddenly, you realize that there is a little person inside there, a new member of your family who is already making their presence felt.

Here is an analogy. Think of the woman's body as a lovingly tended garden, where a seed – your baby – has been planted. It is in that third month when the seed sprouts and begins to grow into a visible plant – the bump, a sign of the miraculous life evolving inside her. Watching this transformation can be like witnessing a sunrise, a slow reveal of something beautiful that fills you with warmth.

There is no denying that this phase can be accompanied by a flurry of mixed emotions. Your partner may grapple with body image issues as her physique alters, sometimes dramatically. As the pregnancy progresses, clothes might stop fitting, activities she once enjoyed might become challenging, and body aches may make her routine difficult.

In such moments, your role as a supportive partner is pivotal. Your reassurances can provide the balm for her anxieties and boost her confidence. Celebrate her transforming body, and remind her of the marvel it is creating. Consider framing it this way, "Each change in your body is a chapter in the story we are writing together. Our baby's story." Every curve, every stretch mark, every kick – they are signs of the love you both are bringing into the world.

It is essential to openly communicate during this period. Ask her how she is feeling, listen to her concerns, and acknowledge her experiences. This empathetic approach will make her feel seen and supported.

A practical tip? Plan a "bump date." Make it a weekly ritual to take pictures of the progressing bump together. This can turn into a beautiful timeline of your journey toward parenthood. Not only will this be a cherished keepsake in years to come, but it will also help you both bond over the shared joy of anticipating your baby.

Your partner may also start to experience physical discomfort due to her growing bump. Offer to massage her aching back, or propose a relaxing spa day. It is not just about relieving her physical discomfort, but also about reminding her that she is not alone on this journey.

Another way to provide comfort is by taking the initiative to adjust her surroundings as per her changing needs. For instance, invest in pregnancy-friendly items, such as a body pillow for better sleep or comfortable maternity wear that accommodates her growing belly.

Remember that while the physical changes are significant, the emotional shift is just as profound. The image of her changing body in the mirror might sometimes clash with the mental picture she has of herself. It is here that your words of affirmation will mean the most. You might say, "I love the way you are embracing these changes. You have never been more beautiful."

Each day of pregnancy is a step closer to meeting your little one. By appreciating her blossoming bump and offering reassurances, you are also expressing your love for the baby growing inside. Cherish the transformation, offer support, and bask in the shared joy of anticipation. After all, each ripple in her silhouette sings a lullaby of the life you are about to welcome.

Extending Support Amid the Risk of Miscarriage

Every pregnancy is a unique journey, filled with anticipation and joy. However, it is also crucial to remember that not every journey follows the path we expect. We are stepping into a delicate subject now, one often cloaked in silence – the risk of miscarriage.

Have you ever walked on a frozen pond, thrilled by the adventure, yet apprehensive about the ice beneath you? In many ways, the fear of miscarriage feels just like that. There is the excitement of stepping into parenthood, countered by the dread of what could go wrong. This is a profound fear that resides in the heart of every expectant parent. Here, your role as a partner reaches new depths, where empathy, patience, and understanding become the pillars of your support system.

A common myth surrounding miscarriage is that it is rare. The reality, however, is startlingly different. Statistics suggest that about 15-20% of confirmed pregnancies end in miscarriage, with the majority occurring in the first trimester. Although this number might seem intimidating, remember that it is not a certainty; it is a risk, and risks are not guarantees.

Understand that your partner might constantly live under the cloud of this fear. Just because you have had a few good weeks, or even after seeing a strong heartbeat in an ultrasound, her anxiety may not dissipate. The reassuring words "You are pregnant" from the doctor are paradoxically also the starting gun for a race of worries.

So, how do you provide support during such a time? Start with empathy. Empathy is not simply understanding what someone else is feeling; it is sharing those feelings. It is the acknowledgment of her fears, letting her know that they are valid, and you are there with her, every step of the way.

Remember that her hormones could magnify her emotions, causing her to oscillate between joy and dread rapidly. During these emotional storms, your steady presence is what she needs. Let your actions speak more than words – a comforting hug, holding her hand or simply sitting with her in silence.

Maintain open lines of communication. Encourage her to express her fears and concerns without judgment. Listen actively and respond gently. Avoid offering solutions unless asked for; most times, she might just need a patient ear to vent.

Moreover, educate yourself about the signs and symptoms of a potential miscarriage – unusual cramping, spotting, or severe back pain. Knowing these signs will not just make you more prepared; it will also provide an additional layer of reassurance to your partner that you are proactively involved in this journey.

Miscarriage, if it happens, is nobody's fault. Neither yours nor hers. Remember that it is a natural event, often an indication that the pregnancy would not have been healthy. Dealing with such a loss can be overwhelming, so consider seeking professional help if needed. Support groups, therapists, or counselors can provide valuable help in navigating through grief.

Lastly, nurture hope. The road might seem bleak, and the fear of loss might overshadow the joy, but hold onto the hope for a healthier tomorrow, a safer journey, and a beautiful beginning.

The fear of miscarriage is a mountain to be climbed, and you are not alone in this trek. Take one step at a time, bolstered by empathy, understanding, and unconditional love. Always remember: In this journey of parenthood, you are a team, scaling highs and lows together, toward the sunrise of a new life.

Promoting Gentle Exercises for Fitness

Picture this scenario: It is a Sunday morning and you are ambling in the park with your partner, hand in hand. You feel the baby bump and smile, wondering about the miracle happening inside. The sun is warm and the sky is azure. Suddenly, your partner sighs and you look over, her face creased with worry. She is thinking about how her body has changed and how her routine has been upended. You squeeze her hand, reminding her that she is not alone. You can be there, not just emotionally but physically too, to encourage her to stay active, healthy, and confident during this beautiful journey.

Gentle exercise during pregnancy is often recommended by healthcare professionals. Its benefits are multifaceted, impacting both the physical and mental well-being of the expectant mother. From improving mood to aiding in easier labor, light workouts can be an indispensable part of the pregnancy journey. And the best part is, you as an expecting father can actively participate, making it a shared endeavor.

Firstly, let us bust a myth: Exercising during pregnancy is not dangerous. It is beneficial, but like anything else, it requires moderation and an understanding of what activities are appropriate. The intensity and type of workouts will naturally change as the pregnancy progresses, and they should always be discussed with a healthcare provider beforehand.

One of the most recommended exercises is walking. It is simple, requires no special equipment, and can be done anywhere. You could make it a ritual, a time when you both get to connect, talk, and enjoy the surroundings. Gradually increase the distance and speed but remember the golden rule: It should feel comfortable and never strain your partner.

Then comes prenatal yoga, which is excellent for flexibility and strength. It also focuses on breath control and mental discipline, which can be useful during labor. As an expecting father, you can either join your partner in these yoga sessions or help her with practice at home. Besides, yoga can be a tool for relaxation for you as well.

Swimming or water workouts can be a boon during the later stages of pregnancy. The water supports the body's weight, reducing strain on the joints while providing resistance for a light cardio workout. You can join your partner in the pool for swimming laps or just enjoy a relaxing float.

Finally, pelvic floor exercises or Kegels are beneficial in preparing for labor and recovering post-childbirth. While this may seem like an exercise only for your partner, you can provide support by learning about these exercises and gently reminding her to practice daily.

Remember, these exercises are not about maintaining a fitness regimen as much as they are about remaining active, reducing discomfort, and enhancing overall well-being during pregnancy. Encourage your partner to listen to her body. If she feels tired or any discomfort, she should stop and rest.

Being involved in your partner's exercise routine is not just about physical support; it is a way of showing your partner that you are in this together. You are not just expecting a child; you are also nurturing your relationship, making it stronger and ready for the beautiful changes ahead. So, tie those shoelaces, roll out the yoga mats, or get the swimsuits ready, and step into this journey of active pregnancy together.

Chapter 5:
Navigating the Emotions of the Fourth Month

Coping With Hormonal Changes During Mid-Pregnancy

In the fourth month of pregnancy, something akin to an emotional tempest can often begin to brew. It is as if Mother Nature, in her infinite wisdom, decided to combine the creation of new life with a roller coaster ride of feelings. It is fascinating, it is moving, and yes, it can also be a bit daunting for the expectant father standing on the sidelines. Let us delve into why these emotional fluctuations happen and how you, as an involved and caring partner, can offer the support your loved one needs.

Have you ever felt caught off guard by your own emotions? Maybe you have had a day where you were inexplicably elated or unusually down without any particular reason. During pregnancy, your partner is likely to experience these emotional swings on a whole new level, largely due to hormonal changes. It is like her body is conducting an orchestra, with hormones playing a symphony of life. Progesterone and estrogen, in particular, take the lead, rising and falling, stirring emotions as they prepare the body for motherhood.

In the face of these mood swings, your partner may at times feel like a ship tossed in a storm. And you, as her steadfast lighthouse, can help guide her through. This begins with understanding and acknowledging what she is experiencing. It is not "just hormones," it is a profound process happening within her that is as beautiful as it is complex.

Now, you might be wondering, "How can I provide the support she needs?" It is all about creating a safe and comforting environment and, more importantly, listening. Listening, in its genuine sense, is more than hearing words; it is understanding the feelings behind those words. You do not need to have all the answers; sometimes, being a sounding board is enough.

Patience is also key. Remember, it is not personal if she becomes irritated or upset. These are temporary emotional ripples in the pond of pregnancy. One effective strategy is to practice mindful breathing together, a technique that can help you both stay calm and focused. Inhale positivity, exhale negativity. Breathe in calm, breathe out stress. This not only helps at the moment but equips you both with a practical tool to navigate any stressors that come your way.

Consider also the power of small acts of kindness. A warm cup of her favorite caffeine-free tea or a surprise note of encouragement can work wonders to lift her spirits. Keep the atmosphere light and nurturing, remind her of the strength she possesses, and let her know it is okay to feel what she is feeling.

Lastly, remember to take care of yourself as well. It is like the safety instructions given before a flight – put on your oxygen mask before helping others. Your well-being is just as crucial, so take the time to do activities that help you relax and stay centered. A balanced duo can better weather the emotional storms together.

These hormonal changes, while challenging, are normal and temporary. They are part of the miraculous symphony of creating new life. By understanding, listening, showing patience, and taking care of both her and yourself, you can turn this stormy phase into a bonding experience that deepens your relationship. Remember, you are not just a bystander in this process; you are an integral part of this beautiful journey toward parenthood.

Nurturing Patience Amid the Turbulence

Imagine you are out on a lake in a small boat. The water's calm surface perfectly mirrors the vast, cloudless sky above. Then, without warning, a storm blows in. Dark clouds roll overhead, winds whip the surface of the water into frothy waves, and lightning cracks the sky. Would you abandon your boat and dive into the turbulent water? Or would you stay aboard, weathering the storm until calm returns?

Just as you would not abandon your boat in a storm, the same resilience is required when navigating your partner's pregnancy, specifically during the fourth month when hormonal changes can intensify. You can view these hormonal shifts like an unexpected squall. They may bring mood swings, bouts of fatigue, and a myriad of physical discomforts for your partner. Your role as the expectant father is to remain patient, steadfast, offering an unwavering source of support.

Now, let us explore practical ways to cultivate patience during these turbulent times.

Practice Active Listening: Patience often starts with understanding. Set aside time each day to talk with your partner about her experiences and feelings. Listen without interruption or the urge to "fix" everything. Active listening shows empathy, which can help defuse tension and enhance your connection during this transformative period.

Develop Emotional Intelligence: Understanding your own emotions can help you navigate your partner's emotional shifts. If you feel frustration rising, take a moment to identify what is causing this reaction. Are you tired? Stressed? Once you recognize your emotional triggers, you can work on strategies to manage them.

Employ Stress-Relieving Activities: Regular exercise, meditation, or pursuing a hobby can provide a much-needed release valve for your stress. These activities give your mind a break and help maintain your emotional balance. They are not an escape from your partner but rather a way to recharge your patience.

Cultivate Gratitude: It is easy to get lost in the sea of changes and challenges. Practicing daily gratitude can help shift your focus from the difficulties to the blessings. Take time each day to reflect on the positive aspects of your partner's pregnancy and your journey to fatherhood.

Be Present: It is tempting to let your mind race ahead to the upcoming months, the impending labor, and how life will change with the baby. However, by focusing too much on the future, you may miss the beauty of the "now." Being present helps you to appreciate the journey and can make it easier to navigate your partner's emotional waves.

Patience is not just about waiting; it is about maintaining a positive attitude while you wait. You can think of these hormonal storms as necessary for bringing new life into the world. So, anchor your patience, keep your eyes on the horizon, and remember: every storm passes, leaving clear skies and calm waters behind. The storms of pregnancy too will pass, replaced by the joy of holding your newborn baby in your arms. The patience and understanding you cultivate now will not only strengthen your relationship with your partner but also serve you well in your journey into fatherhood.

Remember, you are not just weathering the storm; you are navigating toward the beautiful sunrise of parenthood. Your calm presence in these turbulent times can be the buoy that keeps your family afloat. Stay patient, stay supportive, and above all, keep sailing. Your destination is well worth the journey.

Boosting Her Confidence and Self-Esteem

Remember that day you went to work with an unironed shirt and your hair in disarray? How uncomfortable it made you feel? Now, imagine what your partner might be feeling with all the bodily changes and hormones playing up. The pregnancy, with its physical and emotional upheavals, might just amplify such discomfort to an overwhelming extent. The body she had known for years is now changing at a pace she may not comprehend. It is crucial to help your partner navigate this space, ensuring she feels loved, cherished, and, above all, confident.

One of the best ways to support your partner's self-esteem during pregnancy is through genuine and consistent reassurance. Compliment her on her new, fuller shape, the radiant glow, or the maternal aura she exudes. Even if she brushes them off, know that your words are reaching her, making her feel beautiful and adored.

Remember, your words should not be hollow; let them come from your heart. Sincerity, in this case, is the most potent tool in your armory.

Secondly, engage her in conversations that are not only about the pregnancy. Discuss her interests, passions, and plans. Make her realize she is not just a mother-to-be, but also a woman with dreams, abilities, and individuality. This approach will allow her to retain her sense of self, and not feel overshadowed by the upcoming motherhood.

Promoting a healthy lifestyle together is another uplifting activity. Exercise is a proven mood enhancer. However, intense workouts are not recommended during pregnancy. So, why not accompany her for walks in the park or prenatal yoga classes? These activities will not just keep her healthy, but also foster a shared sense of commitment toward the pregnancy, thereby boosting her spirits.

Encourage her to pamper herself too. Be it a spa day, a day out with friends, or just a quiet reading session, any activity that relaxes and rejuvenates her will contribute to her positive self-image. Let her indulge and take care of herself.

One cannot overstate the significance of open communication. Pregnancy might make her susceptible to mood swings, bouts of anxiety, or even bouts of depression. It is essential to create a safe space where she feels comfortable expressing her fears and concerns without judgment. Encourage her to talk, and more importantly, ensure you are there to listen. You do not always need to offer solutions. Sometimes, being heard is all that one seeks.

Also, do not shy away from seeking professional help if the need arises. If she is feeling persistently low, anxious, or disconnected, it might be more than just pregnancy hormones at play. A professional counselor or a mental health expert could provide the necessary guidance and support.

Remember, as her partner, your role is not limited to providing practical assistance. It also involves being emotionally available and supportive. Pregnancy is a shared journey, and while it is her body that is undergoing the transformation, your mental and emotional support can ease her way. By consistently appreciating, reassuring, and supporting her, you can significantly enhance her self-esteem during these challenging yet beautiful months. After all, the woman carrying your child is nothing short of amazing. Let her know it, and let her feel it, every single day.

Dealing With Pregnancy-Related Sexual Issues

Imagine this: Your partner's body is going through noticeable changes, and you are walking on eggshells, not sure whether you can express your desires for intimacy or if it is even safe to engage in sexual activities. Is this you? It is a common concern many expectant fathers face and an absolutely natural part of the pregnancy journey.

As you navigate the uncharted waters of pregnancy, you might find yourself in a sea of questions. And yes, many of those questions revolve around the subject of intimacy during pregnancy. Is it safe for the baby? Will it cause any harm to my partner? The answer to both these questions is generally, "No." In most normal, healthy pregnancies, intimacy, including sexual intercourse, is completely safe. But there are always exceptions and nuances. So, keep the lines of communication with your partner's healthcare provider wide open.

Pregnancy is a time of physical change, and this includes changes in sexual desires. Hormonal fluctuations can lead to increased or decreased libido in expectant mothers. This can be confusing and perhaps even intimidating for both partners. It is essential to acknowledge these changes without judgment, reminding yourself that these are transient phases in your life journey together.

Now, let us debunk some myths. One of the most common fears is that intercourse can harm the baby. The truth is, your baby is well-protected within the womb by the amniotic sac and the strong muscles of the uterus. Additionally, a mucus plug seals the cervix, safeguarding against infections. But remember, each pregnancy is unique and complications can warrant the need to abstain. Always consult with your partner's healthcare provider if you have any concerns.

Let us talk about how to navigate intimacy during this transformative period. Here are some practical tips to guide you:

Communication Is Key: Have open conversations with your partner about how she is feeling physically and emotionally. This will help you understand her needs better and foster a sense of closeness.

Prioritize Comfort: With the progressing pregnancy, certain positions might not be comfortable or safe. Be open to exploring new positions that are comfortable for your partner.

Intimacy Goes Beyond the Physical: Understand that intimacy is not just about sex. It is about emotional connection, too. This might be a time to explore other ways to be intimate, like cuddling, kissing, or simply spending quality time together.

Be Patient: There might be times when your partner might not feel up to it, respect her feelings and give her the space she needs.

Reassure Her: Pregnancy can bring about body image issues in women. Reassure your partner about your love and attraction toward her.

Stay informed. Talk to the healthcare provider about any concerns related to sexual activity during pregnancy. When in doubt, always ask.

Remember, the most important thing during this time is the well-being of your partner and the baby. This is a time of bonding and deepening your connection, not just as partners, but as co-parents. Even as you navigate the complex dynamics of intimacy during pregnancy, remember to tread with sensitivity, respect, and love. It is a team effort, after all, and you are on this journey together.

Chapter 6:
Embarking on the Fifth Month's Journey

Embracing the Excitement and Apprehension of the Gender Reveal

You are in the fifth month, and the moment of revelation is here – the gender reveal of your baby. It is a critical milestone, a grand disclosure that will suddenly make the abstract idea of parenthood tangible. Boy or girl, it does not matter, but it is the realization that there is a little human growing, one who will soon have an identity, that amplifies both joy and anxiety.

Gender reveals can be a beautiful, shared moment with your partner, family, and friends, but they can also bring up mixed emotions. You might feel a rush of excitement, coupled with fear of the unknown. How should you react? What does this mean for your future? How will it influence your role as a father?

First and foremost, acknowledge these emotions. There is no need to feel guilty about having mixed feelings. Pregnancy is a profound journey filled with many unknowns, and it is natural to feel nervous about the future. When we admit our fears and doubts, we are taking the first step toward understanding them.

If you feel a little disappointed or surprised about the baby's gender, it is okay. It is called "gender disappointment," and it is more common than you think. People usually build scenarios in their minds about what life with a baby boy or a girl will be like, and when the reality is different, it can throw them off. Understand that it is a temporary feeling and it does not mean you will love your baby any less.

It is also important to discuss these feelings with your partner. It is a journey for both of you, and you are in this together. If you are excited, share your joy, and if you are nervous, voice your fears. This open communication will only make you stronger as a couple and more prepared for the baby's arrival.

The gender reveal is also an occasion for celebration. Whether it is a small intimate gathering or an extravagant party, it should be about embracing the news with joy. Plan something that suits your style. If you like surprises, let someone else do the organizing. Or, if you are too excited, plan the reveal yourself. Balloons, cakes, confetti – there are countless ways to make the moment memorable.

Remember, it is not about the baby being a boy or a girl, but about the baby being your child. As you pop that balloon or cut that cake, you are not just revealing a gender; you are celebrating the little life you and your partner created.

You can also use this time to start thinking about names. It is a beautiful way to further personalize the experience. Consider family traditions, shared interests, or simply names you love.

Above all, use this time to strengthen your resolve to be the best dad you can be, regardless of whether you are having a son or a daughter. Instead of worrying about what you cannot control, focus on what you can: Raising your child with love, respect, and kindness. Your baby's gender will not change your capacity to love them or your responsibility toward them.

To conclude, this is a significant moment in your journey toward parenthood. It is all right to feel an array of emotions, from joy to fear. Be honest about your feelings, communicate with your partner, and celebrate this wonderful revelation. It is not just about the gender of your baby; it is about the anticipation of a new life – your child's life – that makes this moment so profound.

The Importance and Benefits of Antenatal Classes for Parenting

Let me pose a question to you: Have you ever considered signing up for an antenatal class? If your immediate response was, "No, that is just for moms," you are not alone. Many men believe that antenatal classes are solely for expectant mothers. But here is a game-changing fact: Antenatal classes offer enormous benefits to future fathers too.

To grasp the potential value these classes could add to your parenting journey, let us travel back in time to your school days. Remember when you first sat behind the wheel of a car in Driver's Ed, your instructor guiding you, explaining the intricacies of the road? Antenatal classes work similarly, only this time, the road you are navigating is the journey toward fatherhood, a drive that can sometimes feel as unpredictable as a rush-hour traffic jam.

There is a saying that I find exceptionally fitting: "Knowledge is power." And antenatal classes are essentially power sessions. They equip you with practical information about pregnancy, labor, birth, and early parenting, preparing you for the various challenges you might face as a father.

The topics these classes cover are wide-ranging. They demystify medical procedures, familiarizing you with terms like "episiotomy," "C-section," "epidural," and the many stages of labor. They will teach you about various birth positions and their benefits, allowing you to be a helpful advocate for your partner during labor. Understanding these aspects can help you support your partner more effectively, providing reassurance and empathy during those stressful times.

Furthermore, they will guide you on newborn care, discussing diaper changing, bathing, swaddling, breastfeeding support, and recognizing signs of common newborn conditions. After all, being a father is not just about emotional support; it is about getting down to the nitty-gritty of practical care, and yes, that includes diaper duty.

One of the most significant aspects of these classes is the opportunity they provide for open discussion. These classes are often filled with couples just like you – eager, excited, and perhaps a little overwhelmed. Engaging with others in a similar stage of life can foster a sense of camaraderie, a reassurance that you are not alone on this journey.

Now, take a moment and envision yourself in a few months. Your partner is in labor, the contractions are coming fast and strong, and the hospital staff is bustling around you. In that intense moment, would you rather be floundering in confusion or equipped with knowledge, ready to provide support?

To find an antenatal class, start with a simple online search or ask your healthcare provider for recommendations. There are various formats available, from in-person classes to online courses, catering to different schedules and comfort levels.

But remember, antenatal classes are not about achieving a "perfect" birth experience or becoming an "expert" in newborn care overnight. Instead, it is about feeling empowered, prepared, and ready to embrace your role as a father. So, I encourage you to take the plunge, sign up for an antenatal class, and start your educational journey into fatherhood. Believe me, the benefits will be well worth the investment.

Strategizing for a Financially Secure Future

"Congratulations, you are going to be a dad!" is undoubtedly one of the most beautiful sentences you will ever hear in your life. But as you are swept up in this whirlwind of emotions, a lingering question might start to creep in – how are you going to afford this?

Welcoming a new baby into your life is not just emotionally transformative; it is financially transformative too. So how do you pivot from panicking about pennies to confidently providing for your growing family? Let us tackle this together, step by step.

Firstly, begin by understanding that having a baby will indeed affect your finances. This is not intended to scare you, but to prepare you. When you acknowledge this reality, you are already a step ahead.

The next step is to review your current financial situation. Get an overview of your income, expenses, and savings. How much do you earn? What are your regular expenses? How much do you manage to save each month? These figures will serve as your foundation for the financial planning ahead.

Once you have got a clear picture, it is time to start budgeting for the baby. A few significant costs you will need to factor in include prenatal care, the cost of childbirth, postnatal care, and the daily expenses of raising a child. These might include baby food, clothing, diapers, and healthcare, not to mention larger one-time expenses like a crib, a stroller, and a car seat.

Here is where your previously identified savings come into play. It would be wise to allocate a portion of these savings toward these upcoming expenses. Consider opening a separate savings account specifically for this purpose.

And do not forget about health insurance. Scrutinize your existing policy to see what maternity and pediatric coverage it offers. You may need to adjust your policy or look into additional coverage options to ensure your partner and baby's medical needs will be adequately covered.

But financial planning does not stop at just budgeting and insurance. One crucial aspect often overlooked is planning for maternity and paternity leave. Depending on your employment situation, you and your partner may receive paid leave, or it might be partially paid, or not paid at all. It is essential to understand your rights and your employer's policies so you can budget for this period of reduced income.

Planning financially for a baby might seem like a daunting task, but it does not have to be. By breaking it down into manageable steps – understanding the costs involved, reviewing your financial situation, budgeting carefully, ensuring adequate insurance, and planning for parental leave – you are well on your way to ensuring a secure future for your family.

Take it from millions of parents who have walked this path before: Yes, kids are expensive, but they are worth every penny. So take a deep breath, put pen to paper, and start preparing for the incredible journey of fatherhood that lies ahead. You have got this!

Fostering a Bond With the Baby Through the Power of Touch

Picture this: You are seated next to your partner, your hand resting on her growing belly. Suddenly, you feel a tiny push from within, a small blip under your palm. It is your unborn child, responding to your touch, affirming their presence. This magical moment is the beginning of a bond that can only deepen with time.

As an expecting father, you might feel somewhat sidelined during pregnancy as all the physical changes are happening to your partner. But remember, you too have an important role in this journey. Your baby can hear you, feel your touch, and even react to it. That is incredible, do you agree? Your bond with your child starts now, right in the womb, and it begins with something as simple yet profound as touch.

Talking and singing to your unborn child is wonderful and it fosters an early connection. But it is the act of touching that makes the bonding experience more tangible. It is an intimate communication, one that speaks of love, protection, and anticipation. The key is to be present, patient, and intentional in these moments.

Start with simple actions. Lay your hand gently on your partner's belly. Feel the smooth roundness, the warmth of the life within. It is your baby, growing and thriving. These quiet moments of contact can be a soothing routine, perhaps before bed when everything is peaceful, and it is just you, your partner, and your baby.

Next, experiment with a light massage. Not only does this make your partner feel loved and relaxed, but it also lets your baby know that you are there. Remember to check with your partner to ensure the pressure is comfortable. Use this time to talk to your baby, to let them know about their daddy who is eagerly waiting to meet them.

And then, await the magic. The kicks, the rolls, the pushes. These are your baby's replies to your touch. It is their way of saying, "Hi, Daddy, I can feel you too." In these moments, you are not an outsider. You are an integral part of this extraordinary journey.

Do not worry if your baby does not respond immediately or every time. Just like us, babies have sleep cycles and quieter moments. What matters is the consistency of your attempts to connect.

Importantly, respect your partner's boundaries and comfort. Pregnancy can bring about sensitivity and discomfort, so always communicate and check in with her before touching the baby bump.

Your journey toward fatherhood is paved with these beautiful, shared moments of anticipation and connection. These initial interactions, these soft whispers of love, create a bridge between you and your unborn child. They form the foundation of your future relationship, a bond that is nurtured in the womb and blossoms in the world.

So, take these moments and hold them close. Let the power of touch guide you on this path. You are not just becoming a father; you are already one. Cherish this time, for it is fleeting, and it is precious.

Remember, every touch, every word, every loving look toward your partner's belly is a step closer to your baby.

Can you feel it? The thrill of connection, the stirrings of love? That is your baby, reaching out, bonding with you. Embrace it, nurture it, and let it grow, just like your child. These moments, fleeting as they may be, are the beginning of a lifetime of love and connection. You are on this journey together, every step of the way.

Cultivating a Supportive Community of Prepared Fathers

As men venturing into the exhilarating world of pregnancy and parenthood, we often find ourselves feeling lost or overwhelmed, even if we are brimming with excitement. There are moments when we might feel like we are the only ones struggling to navigate this complex journey.

Yet, rest assured, there are countless fathers out there feeling exactly the same way. My aim with this book is not only to provide you with a practical guide through the intricate phases of pregnancy but also to remind you that you are part of an expansive community of men evolving into first-time dads. Your experiences, emotions, and uncertainties are shared by many.

And here is an easy way for you to lend a helping hand to others on the same journey – it will require just a few minutes of your time but could significantly influence another man's path into fatherhood.

By leaving an honest review of this book on Amazon, you will be contributing invaluable insights to potential readers. Your experience with this guide can shine a light on its value and its capacity to assist. You will be extending a reassuring hand to other men, letting them know they are not alone and that this resource can help guide them through the journey.

Providing this feedback will not just help them discover a supportive resource, it will also build a sense of solidarity among us, affirming that we are all traversing the same path, facing the same challenges, and celebrating the same victories.

Scan to leave a review !

Remember, your input is important. Whether positive or constructive, your feedback assists in shaping future editions of this book and serves as a beacon for others venturing into fatherhood.

Your contribution helps build a community. Let us lift each other as we embark on the wonderful journey of becoming fathers.

Thank you in advance for your support. As we progress into fatherhood, remember, together, we can foster a well-prepared and supportive community of dads.

Chapter 7:
Unveiling the Peaceful Oasis of the Sixth Month

Alleviating Her Pregnancy Discomfort With Massage Therapy

Can you recall the first time your partner shared her pregnancy news? It was a unique feeling, right? A myriad of emotions played at that moment. Since then, you have accompanied her through a wonderful, yet complex journey, in which every day is a new chapter. Now, as you have stepped into the sixth month, the story takes a slight turn. The plot thickens as your partner begins to experience physical discomforts – backaches, swelling, and the like. Fear not, for you have a secret weapon at your disposal – the power of touch.

You might be thinking, "I am not a massage therapist!" True, but believe it or not, you can play an integral role in soothing these discomforts. Pregnancy massage is not only a therapeutic technique but also a unique opportunity to deepen your bond with your partner and the unborn baby. In this section, we will explore how you can provide effective pregnancy massages and turn these moments into meaningful bonding sessions.

Let us start with the basics. Pregnancy massage is a specialized form of massage designed to alleviate physical discomforts caused by pregnancy changes. It focuses on areas such as the back, legs, and feet, which commonly suffer from tension or swelling. Do not worry; you do not need to be an expert to do this! Remember, the intention here is not to give a professional-grade massage but to offer comfort and reassurance through your touch.

Here is how you can proceed: Start by creating a tranquil atmosphere; play soothing music, dim the lights, and ensure the room is warm. Encourage your partner to lie on her side, supporting her belly with a cushion. Use a gentle yet firm touch, and apply a safe-for-pregnancy massage oil for a smoother experience.

Beginning with her neck and shoulders, use your fingers and palms to apply gentle pressure, making small circles. Gradually work your way down to the back, keeping communication open. Ask her about the pressure, and adjust accordingly. This simple back massage technique can do wonders for relieving pregnancy-induced backaches.

To address swelling, particularly in the feet and ankles, use a different approach. Elevate her feet and apply gentle strokes moving upwards toward the heart. This encourages blood flow and reduces swelling.

Now, while the physical benefits are apparent, the emotional benefits are profound. As you guide your hands across her body, you are silently communicating your support. This act serves as a physical manifestation of your emotional backing, providing reassurance to her during this journey. Each touch conveys a simple yet powerful message – "I am here with you."

By engaging in pregnancy massage, you are doing much more than alleviating physical discomfort. You are stepping into the world of shared experiences, reinforcing your bond with your partner, and forming an indirect connection with your unborn baby. You are actively participating in the pregnancy, making it a shared journey rather than a solo endeavor.

The power of touch is incredible. Remember, the key here is patience, empathy, and open communication. Use these as your guiding principles while giving pregnancy massages, and you will not only ease her discomfort but also deepen your relationship in the process.

This journey might seem complex and confusing, but is also beautifully unique. As you traverse this path with your partner, every small act you perform, every little comfort you provide, each shared laughter or soothing massage – they all add up, creating a journey that is uniquely yours. And that, dear reader, is the essence of becoming a father.

Creating a Tranquil Nursery for Your Little One

Remember that moment of exhilaration when you held that freshly painted miniature chair? Or when you found the perfect moon-and-stars mobile that matched the nursery theme? Putting together your baby's nursery is a labor of love, infused with dreams, anticipation, and perhaps a little bit of nesting instinct too. It is more than just a room; it is the space where your little one will grow, learn, play, and create memories that will last a lifetime.

First, let us talk about the essentials. Every nursery needs a crib or bassinet, a changing table, a dresser for clothes, and a comfortable chair for feeding or soothing the baby to sleep. Safety comes first in choosing these items. Ensure that the crib slats are close enough together to keep the baby safe, and secure heavy furniture to the wall to prevent tipping. Opt for a changing table with straps and sides that are raised to prevent any rolling incidents.

Next, consider the layout. Keep the crib away from windows to avoid drafts and possible safety hazards like blind cords. Place the changing table near the diaper supply for convenience. And make sure that your comfortable chair has a good light source nearby for those middle-of-the-night feedings or story sessions.

Decorating the nursery can be a delightful process. Choosing a theme or color palette can give the room a cohesive feel. Soft, muted tones or warm neutrals are popular choices, as they create a serene and calming environment. A favorite children's book, a hobby, or even a sweet animal motif can serve as inspiration for your theme. The key is to create a space that feels inviting and comforting, not just for the baby, but for you as well.

Remember, this is your chance to put your stamp on the room. Personalize it! Hang family photos or artworks, perhaps even some of your own childhood mementos. You could also include a special corner for siblings to feel involved. A little shelf with books and toys dedicated for when they visit their new brother or sister could help ease the transition and promote bonding.

Preparing the nursery is also about preparing for the practical aspects of parenting. Think about storage. Babies come with a lot of gear, and you will need places to store clothes, diapers, toys, and books. Use baskets, bins, and shelves to keep everything organized and easily accessible.

Now, imagine standing in the doorway of your completed nursery. It is a tranquil oasis, a labor of love prepared by two people eagerly awaiting their new arrival. Each piece of furniture, every decoration, and even the organization serve a purpose – to create a safe, serene, and loving environment for your child.

Creating a nursery is an incredible bonding experience. It is about more than just paint colors and furniture placements; it is a tangible representation of your love and anticipation for your baby. Every choice you make in setting up this room is a step toward welcoming your child into a home filled with love and warmth. As you look around at the room you have created, let it serve as a reminder of the incredible journey that you and your partner are embarking on together.

Remember, this room is just the beginning. It is the first of many beautiful spaces you will create for your child, filled with love, laughter, and cherished memories. So, take a moment, stand back, and admire your work. The countdown to your baby's arrival just got a little more real. And you are ready.

Finding Common Ground on Parenting Strategies

Can you recall those long-standing debates with your partner about whether pineapple is an acceptable pizza topping or if the toilet roll should go over or under? Suddenly, they might seem insignificant when placed next to the debates you will now face: "How should we raise our child?"

Indeed, as parents-to-be, it is crucial to have open and respectful discussions about your parenting philosophies long before the baby arrives. These dialogues provide the platform to align your parenting strategies, identify potential areas of conflict, and establish mutual respect for differing perspectives. Let us dive into how you can approach these conversations effectively.

Firstly, start the conversation on a positive note. Try to frame it as a journey you both are undertaking together, rather than a negotiation where one must win or lose. A simple conversation starter could be, "I am so excited about this parenting journey we are embarking on. I think it would be great to discuss how we envision raising our child. What do you think?"

When discussing your parenting styles, it is imperative to understand that it is okay to have different views. Remember, your opinions are shaped by your upbringing, past experiences, and individual beliefs. Respect each other's perspectives and aim to find common ground. The goal is not to create a clone of your parents or rebel against their techniques entirely but to foster a nurturing environment for your baby that aligns with your collective values.

Active listening is another essential component of these conversations. When your partner is sharing their thoughts, listen to understand rather than respond. Acknowledge their feelings and concerns, and then share your perspective. A statement like, "I understand where you are coming from, and here is what I think ..." promotes open dialogue and mutual respect.

Now, what topics should you be discussing? There are countless parenting decisions to ponder, from your approach to discipline and setting boundaries to your attitudes about education and societal norms. It is also worth discussing how you will share parenting duties, how to handle disagreements in front of the child, and what values you wish to instill. Remember, the idea is not to have a detailed script but to create an open line of communication.

Despite all the planning and discussion, remember that it is okay not to have everything figured out. Parenting is a journey filled with unexpected twists and turns. You and your partner will continually learn, adapt, and grow as parents, and your philosophies may evolve along the way.

Keep in mind that these conversations are not a one-time thing. They should be ongoing discussions, adapting as your child grows and new situations arise. Perhaps you may also consider engaging in parenting workshops or classes together, where you can gain new insights and discuss them further in your own time.

At the heart of these discussions, remember why you are having them in the first place: Your unwavering love for the baby that is soon to come. As long as that love remains the foundation of your parenting journey, you both will navigate through any disagreements or challenges that come your way. You are in this together, every step of the way.

Navigating these conversations might seem challenging, but they are a vital part of your co-parenting journey. Remember, open dialogue, active listening, respect for differing views, and a willingness to adapt are key. It is about laying a solid foundation for your shared journey into parenthood.

Getting Emotionally Ready for the Arrival of the New Life

Remember that moment when you first found out you were going to be a father? You might have felt a rush of emotions – excitement, joy, and perhaps even a hint of trepidation. As the due date looms, these feelings may intensify, leaving you oscillating between anticipation and apprehension. It is okay to admit that becoming a parent can feel a bit like standing on the edge of an unknown precipice.

In this critical stage, your mind might be swirling with "What ifs." What if something goes wrong during the birth? What if I am not a good dad? What if I cannot balance work and fatherhood? What if … It is completely normal to have these thoughts. After all, you are about to step into a significant new role that comes with enormous responsibility.

However, it is crucial not to let these anxieties overtake your journey. To help manage them, consider the following strategies:

Open Up About Your Fears: First and foremost, remember that you are not alone in this. Your partner likely shares some of these apprehensions too. Talking about your feelings with her can bring relief and create a space for mutual support. If needed, reach out to friends who are already fathers. Their experiences and advice can help you see things from a different perspective.

Practice Mindfulness: Engage in mindfulness exercises, like meditation or deep breathing, to maintain a calm mind. Mindfulness helps anchor you to the present, freeing your mind from anxiety-inducing thoughts about the future.

Stay Active: Regular physical activity is known to reduce stress levels. Whether it is a brisk walk, a gym session, or simply playing a sport you love, keep your body moving. Physical exercise releases endorphins – your body's natural mood boosters.

Prepare, Do Not Panic: Instead of worrying about what might go wrong, channel your energy into preparations. Read parenting books, attend prenatal classes, prepare the baby's room, or take an infant CPR class. These activities not only keep you productive but also give you a sense of control over the situation.

Remember, it is perfectly okay to seek professional help if anxiety begins to affect your daily life. Consult with a mental health professional who can guide you through these feelings.

Also, cherish these moments. The final stretch of your partner's pregnancy is a unique phase, one marked by anticipation and emotional bonding with your unborn child. Try to appreciate the beauty of these moments amid the natural anxiety that comes with them.

Embrace the emotional journey just as much as the physical one. While it is true that becoming a parent is a giant leap into the unknown, it is also the most rewarding journey you will ever embark on. Let the love for your unborn child guide you, giving you the strength to face any fear that comes your way.

Your emotions, no matter how complex or overwhelming, are all a part of this incredible journey called parenthood. Remember, courage does not mean the absence of fear, but the triumph over it. Let this be your mantra as you count down the days to the grand arrival of your little one.

Chapter 8:
Crafting the Seventh Month's Symphony

Connecting With the Unborn Baby Through Your Voice

Picture this: You are sitting comfortably on your favorite couch with a hand resting gently on your partner's burgeoning belly. You are sharing your day, humming a soothing melody, or perhaps even reading from a well-loved book. You are not just sharing a peaceful moment with your partner; you are also communicating with your unborn child.

Many studies have shown that the unborn baby begins to hear and recognize sounds as early as the 20th week of pregnancy. The sound that resonates most? The constant, rhythmic beat of their mother's heart and the muffled cadence of her voice. However, nestled within these familiar and comforting sounds is also room for another – the father's voice.

Although it may seem incredible, your unborn child can indeed learn to distinguish your voice while still in the womb. When you consistently talk to your baby, you are not merely providing them with auditory experiences; you are laying the groundwork for a bond that will continue to grow once your child is born.

Consider this as your first introduction to your child, an opportunity to build familiarity and connection, even before you meet face-to-face. From a practical standpoint, speaking or singing to your unborn baby is as simple as it sounds. However, if you are wondering how to go about it, here are some practical tips.

First, find a quiet space where you can be close to your partner and your unborn child. This could be at the end of the day when you are both unwinding or perhaps a dedicated time you set aside specifically for this purpose.

Begin with a gentle, comforting voice. You do not have to follow a script – talk about your day, your hopes for your child, or share stories of your childhood. The content is not as critical as the consistency and the emotional warmth you convey. Even reading out loud from a book or singing a soft tune can be incredibly beneficial.

This practice offers several advantages, both for you as expectant parents and for your baby. For one, your voice, alongside the mother's, becomes a source of comfort and familiarity for your child. Post-birth, this can significantly help in soothing a crying baby or getting them to sleep. It also aids in the baby's cognitive development, with research showing that babies who were exposed to conversation in utero showed superior language skills.

Moreover, this practice is not just beneficial for the baby; it is advantageous for the expectant father too. At times, the physical disconnect between an expectant father and the unborn child can feel rather overwhelming. Talking or singing to the unborn child helps bridge that gap, creating a tangible connection between the two. It is a ritual that gives you time to comprehend the approaching reality of fatherhood, helping alleviate anxiety or fear about the impending change.

In essence, the simple act of talking or singing to your unborn child becomes an enriching journey of bonding, growth, and anticipation for the miracle that is yet to come. This connection you are nurturing now will echo throughout your child's life, reflecting in their attachment to you and their overall emotional and cognitive development.

As you navigate this journey, remember to give yourself grace. Speaking to your unborn child might feel strange initially, but as with all things related to parenthood, it becomes more comfortable with practice and patience. The key lies in persistence, love, and the knowledge that your voice is not just a sound to your unborn child; it is the beginning of a lifelong bond.

Baby Showers – A Time to Celebrate Your Unborn Child

Have you ever attended a baby shower? It is a festive event filled with joy, laughter, and anticipation of the new life to come. But as a soon-to-be-dad, your role at this party may not be as clear-cut as it would be if you were just a guest. While traditionally seen as an event for mothers, baby showers have evolved to become more inclusive, inviting fathers to be a part of this special celebration. In this section, we will explore the role you can play in your baby shower, how to manage your expectations, and how to contribute to a meaningful and memorable experience for all involved.

Baby showers serve a dual purpose. They are not only about celebrating the forthcoming birth but also preparing the expectant parents with essential items for their baby. While your partner might be more focused on the decoration, theme, or cake design, your attention might be more needed in other aspects. For example, you can help by managing the guest list, setting up the gift registry, or even planning some fun games.

Remember that your role in the baby shower is not to overshadow your partner, but rather to offer your support, and share in the joy and anticipation of your baby's arrival. The event can be a vital space for you to share your excitement, fears, and hopes about fatherhood with friends and family. You might be surprised by how much sharing and learning can happen over a slice of cake!

Managing expectations can be another challenging part of baby showers. While it is an occasion to receive gifts for your newborn, it is essential to maintain a genuine attitude of gratitude. Understand that people might have different budgets and some may opt for handmade or sentimental gifts. Do not let the size or price of the gifts set your mood for the day. Remember, it is the thought that counts.

Planning or participating in a baby shower can seem overwhelming, but it does not have to be. Here are some practical tips:

Work as a Team: Coordinate with your partner to divide responsibilities based on your interests and skills. For instance, if you are tech-savvy, you can handle the digital aspects like online invitations or virtual broadcasting of the event for distant relatives and friends.

Include Other Dads: If you have friends who are fathers, invite them. They can share their experiences, provide practical advice, and perhaps some fatherhood jokes!

Get Involved in Games: Baby shower games are not just for the ladies. Participate, or even suggest a game that you and your buddies can enjoy.

Have a Say in the Registry: Ensure you have a part in creating the gift registry. After all, you are also going to be using those baby items.

Say "Thank You": A simple "thank you" goes a long way. People love knowing that their gifts and presence are appreciated.

Remember, every celebration is about creating beautiful memories, and a baby shower is no different. Your active participation not only makes the event more enjoyable but also deepens your connection with your partner, your baby, and the shared joy of the upcoming new chapter in your life. It is all about celebrating love, growth, and the fantastic journey of parenting you are about to embark upon.

Preparing Yourself for the Childbirth Experience

Picture this scenario: A man, hair frazzled, eyes wide, standing in a hospital hallway while his partner is in the delivery room. Sounds familiar? It is a common trope in movies. But what if I told you that this is not the role you are destined to play? The birth of your child is not a moment where you are sidelined, rather, it is your chance to step up and be a rock for your partner in a moment of intense vulnerability and transformation.

Childbirth, as beautiful and miraculous as it is, can also be nerve-wracking, not only for the mother but also for you, the soon-to-be father. It is unpredictable and can be lengthy, with potential complications that can set your heart racing. Understanding the process can help you be a source of strength and reassurance to your partner, and participate actively in welcoming your baby into the world.

Childbirth happens in three stages. The first is labor, where contractions help dilate the cervix to about 10 centimeters. This stage can take several hours, especially in first pregnancies. The second stage is delivery, where your partner will push the baby through the birth canal. The third and final stage is the delivery of the placenta, an organ that provided nourishment to your baby.

Some complications that could arise include prolonged labor, breech birth (where the baby is positioned feet or bottom first), or the need for an emergency C-section. These may sound scary, but remember that medical professionals are trained to handle these situations. You can equip yourself with knowledge to better understand these situations, but ultimately, trust in the expertise of the doctors and midwives present.

Your role in the delivery room is multifaceted. First and foremost, you provide emotional support. It is not just about holding your partner's hand, but also about helping her stay calm and focused, reminding her to breathe and relax, encouraging her, and being there for her in any way she needs. This could mean massaging her back, getting her ice chips, or even just being a reassuring presence.

Secondly, you will be a communication link between your partner and the medical team. Your partner will be busy concentrating on her labor. If you have discussed a birth plan, you can help communicate her preferences to the team, like positions she wants to try or if she wants to avoid certain medications.

Lastly, be prepared for practical tasks. This could be anything from timing contractions at home before heading to the hospital, packing a hospital bag with all necessary items, to filling out the necessary paperwork.

Remember, childbirth is not a spectator sport. It is a team effort. Staying informed, calm, supportive, and actively involved can help you transform from a frazzled, sidelined participant to an empowered, supportive partner in the birthing process. This is not just about making the experience less stressful for your partner, but also about participating in one of life's most profound moments - the birth of your child. You are not just an onlooker; you are a key player in this beautiful symphony of life. So brace yourself, for this is a moment you will remember and cherish forever.

Prioritizing Mother and Baby's Well-Being With Regular Health Check-Ups

Do you remember the first time you held your partner's hand during a doctor's visit? Recall the mixture of anticipation and anxiety as you walked through those hospital doors together. Now, as you navigate the final stretch of pregnancy, those prenatal check-ups in the third trimester have become an indispensable part of your journey. This is where you gain precious insights into the well-being of your partner and your soon-to-be child, where you uncover any potential complications before they escalate, and where you learn to ask the right questions to empower your partner and yourself.

It is essential to remember that these visits are not just a routine. Each appointment serves as a touchpoint, an opportunity to reassess and recalibrate. With every heartbeat monitored and every ultrasound examined, the picture of your baby's health becomes more transparent, enabling doctors to spot any irregularities or concerns promptly. It is your duty, as an expectant father, to become a proficient interpreter of this information, not just a passive observer. So, make sure to ask questions, lots of them. Do not let any jargon bewilder you. Ask for clarifications. Ask for explanations. Remember, knowledge is power, and this power will help you support your partner better.

At each appointment, doctors will monitor your partner's health – her blood pressure, weight, and more – while also checking on the baby's development. There will be discussions about labor signs and the various stages of labor. Remember, these are not one-way conversations. Your role here is not just to listen but to participate actively. The doctors are there to provide guidance, but you are the one accompanying your partner in this journey, so your understanding and engagement matter.

Understanding the significance of these tests is vital. For example, the "Group B Strep test," usually done between 35 to 37 weeks of pregnancy, checks for bacteria that could potentially be harmful to the baby during childbirth. If positive, your partner would need antibiotics during labor to protect the baby. Grasping such information can prevent unnecessary panic if the situation arises.

Often, prospective fathers feel like they are on a sideline, watching as a spectator rather than participating. However, your presence and support during these check-ups can significantly impact your partner's comfort and stress levels. Engage with the healthcare provider, be attentive, and most importantly, be empathetic.

One of the questions you could ask during these visits is about recognizing signs of preterm labor. It is crucial to know when it is time to rush to the hospital or when it is a false alarm. Inquire about the hospital's policies on birthing plans, visitation rules, and pain management options during labor. All this information can help you prepare a contingency plan, reducing the chances of panic when the big day arrives.

To sum it up, these health check-ups are an essential component of your journey toward fatherhood. They are the opportunities that allow you to transition from an expectant father to an informed and proactive co-parent. The path may be overwhelming, but remember, it is a shared journey. You are not just an observer; you are a partner. Make the most out of each visit, ask questions, get involved, and support your partner every step of the way.

The magical day when you hold your baby for the first time is just around the corner. Be prepared, be informed, and be present. After all, every journey is more manageable when navigated together.

Chapter 9:
Immersing in the Eighth Month's Prelude

Offering Support Through Late Pregnancy Challenges

Imagine for a moment that you are carrying a weight; a beautiful, precious weight that grows heavier each day. It tugs at your back, pushes against your ribs, and disrupts your sleep. That is what the last trimester of pregnancy can feel like for many women. As a soon-to-be dad, it is your job to understand these challenges and find ways to help.

The eighth month of pregnancy is a mix of anticipation and discomfort. Your partner may find it increasingly difficult to get a good night's sleep. Her back might be aching from the strain of carrying the baby. She may frequently feel out of breath, even with minimal activity. While this can be a trying time, remember that every challenge presents an opportunity for you to step up and support her.

First, let us address sleep disturbances. These often stem from the baby's size, making it difficult for the mother to find a comfortable sleeping position. An effective way to help is by investing in a pregnancy pillow. These pillows are designed to support the curves of the pregnant body, providing comfort and promoting better sleep. You can also encourage her to sleep on her left side, as this position improves circulation to the heart, benefiting both mom and baby.

Next, there is the backache. As the baby grows, it places additional pressure on the mother's lower back, often leading to pain. Offering a gentle massage can provide immense relief. Keep in mind that the massage should be gentle, focusing on relaxing the muscles rather than deep tissue work. Encourage her to communicate what feels good and where she needs the most relief. If you are unsure, consider booking a professional massage therapist who specializes in prenatal care.

Shortness of breath is another common challenge. The growing baby puts pressure on the diaphragm, making it harder for the lungs to expand fully. Assure your partner that this is common and encourage slow, deep breaths. Setting aside quiet moments for deep breathing exercises can help increase her lung capacity and reduce anxiety.

Importantly, remind her to take it easy. The chores can wait; the world will not end if the house is a bit messy. Offer to take over some tasks and encourage her to rest often.

Lastly, be proactive in helping her stay hydrated and maintain a balanced diet. Nutritious food and plenty of fluids can help alleviate many discomforts, including fatigue and constipation.

Supporting your partner during this time is not just about easing her physical discomforts, though. The final trimester can be a whirlwind of emotions, from excitement to apprehension. Talk to her, reassure her of your love and support, and share in the joy and anticipation of meeting your little one soon.

Remember, this is not just about survival, it is about thriving together. This is a time of deep connection and growth for you both.

By understanding and addressing these challenges, you are laying the foundation for a stronger relationship and a stronger family.

And hey, who knew a dad could be a master of massages, a connoisseur of comfort foods, and a wizard of soothing words all at once? Rise to the occasion, future dads. Your partners and your babies are worth every moment of it.

Making Sure You Are a Part of the Birth Plan

Do you remember that time when you meticulously planned your vacation? You read every guidebook, researched every travel forum, and poured over maps until you could navigate the city like a local. That is exactly the level of preparation you need as you step into your role in the birth plan. It is not just about being present in the delivery room; it is about being actively involved in the decisions that affect your partner and your baby.

So, how do you, as an expectant father, contribute to the birth plan effectively? First, let us understand what a birth plan is. It is a document that communicates your partner's wishes for the labor and delivery process. It addresses aspects like pain management, birthing positions, who is present during birth, and preferences for handling any unexpected situations. It is not set in stone but acts as a guide, a point of discussion with the healthcare provider.

Having a plan does not mean you are demanding a specific course of action. Rather, it is about expressing preferences and preparing for various scenarios. It is about ensuring your partner feels heard and respected. This is where you come in. Your role is not just to support your partner, but also to ensure that her wishes are communicated and understood by the healthcare team.

To contribute effectively, start by familiarizing yourself with the birthing process. Read up on different pain management techniques, from epidurals to natural methods like hypnobirthing or water birth. Learn about birthing positions and their benefits. Know the difference between a routine intervention and an emergency one. Knowledge is power, and in this case, it can lead to a more positive birthing experience.

Once you are informed, initiate discussions with your partner. Encourage her to express her fears and wishes. Remember, these conversations might be emotionally charged, and your partner may have strong feelings about certain issues. Respect her views and provide comfort and reassurance. Your empathetic tone will provide her with a sense of security knowing that you are in this together.

When creating the birth plan, consider writing it together. This shared experience not only makes you an active participant but also strengthens your bond as a couple. Use a collaborative tool or a simple piece of paper, and write down your preferences. Seeing your thoughts on paper can help you both understand and respect each other's perspectives better.

Keep in mind that the birth plan should be flexible. Labor and delivery can be unpredictable, and sometimes medical interventions are necessary for the safety of the mother and the baby. So, while it is crucial to have preferences, it is equally important to trust the expertise of the healthcare provider and be open to changes if needed.

Finally, be the advocate for your partner during labor and delivery. You may need to communicate her wishes to the medical team, especially during intense moments. By being knowledgeable, confident, and calm, you can be the pillar of support she needs.

Remember, the birth plan is not a test you pass or fail. It is about making an uncertain situation slightly more predictable and ensuring that your partner's birthing experience aligns as closely as possible with her wishes. By being involved in this process, you are showing your commitment to her and your soon-to-be-born child.

Embarking on a D-Day Hospital Tour

Have you ever tried to navigate an unfamiliar city without a map? You would likely end up frustrated, lost, and late to your destination. Consider the hospital tour as your "map" to the delivery day; it is your golden ticket to be prepared, calm, and supportive when your partner needs you the most.

Before we delve into the why's and what's of a hospital tour, remember that this is a shared journey. Encourage your partner to accompany you on the hospital tour. This shared experience will not only provide her with a sense of familiarity and comfort but will also allow both of you to ask questions and clarify your doubts.

Let us start with the why's. Why should you embark on a hospital tour? First and foremost, a hospital tour is an invaluable source of information. It is an opportunity to become acquainted with the physical layout of the hospital – where to park, where to register, where the birthing suites are located, and, crucially, where to go on the day of delivery. The last thing you want to be doing while your partner is in labor is to be wandering around the hospital in confusion.

On this tour, you will also gain insight into the hospital's approach to labor and delivery. Every hospital has its own protocol. Some might have labor, delivery, recovery, and postpartum (LDRP) rooms where the entire birth process takes place in one room. Others may transfer mothers and newborns from one room to another. Understanding this process can significantly alleviate stress and confusion on the big day.

Furthermore, familiarizing yourself with the hospital's policies is essential. Will you be allowed in the delivery room if your partner opts for a C-section? Can you bring a camera to capture the first few moments of your baby's life? Are there any restrictions on visitors? Knowledge of these policies will equip you to plan better and manage expectations.

A hospital tour also provides a glimpse into the support and facilities available. Birthing suites may vary in terms of equipment like birthing balls, stools, and squatting bars. Is there an option for water birth? What kind of pain management options are available? These details can be vital in finalizing your birth plan.

So, you now understand the importance of a hospital tour. But what can you do to make the most of it? Firstly, be proactive. Do not hesitate to ask questions, no matter how trivial they might seem. Remember, this tour is for you to gather as much information as possible.

Next, take notes or photos (if allowed). These can act as valuable references as you prepare for D-Day. You might think you will remember everything, but amid the excitement and anticipation, details can easily be forgotten.

Lastly, pay attention to the atmosphere and the staff. Your partner's comfort is paramount, and an empathetic and supportive team can make a world of difference to her birth experience.

Consider this as a reconnaissance mission. You are gathering essential information to make the birth of your child a seamless and joyous experience. Each step you take in familiarizing yourself with the hospital environment is a step toward reducing uncertainty and building confidence for the upcoming arrival of your little one. Remember, knowledge is power. Equip yourself with it, and you will be a pillar of strength for your partner on the day your lives change forever.

Preparing With Assembled Baby Gear

Imagine this: The delivery day is finally here. You are elated, a little nervous, but ready to meet your little one. You and your partner get to the car, and you suddenly realize that the car seat is still in its box, unassembled. At that moment, the anxiety of setting it up correctly, not to mention the pressure of time, can turn into a truly stressful situation. Let us prevent this from happening.

Starting with the car seat, it is essential to remember that this is not just a regular seat. It is a safety device designed to protect the most precious cargo you will ever carry. When shopping for one, look for those approved by the safety standards in your country. Once you have selected and bought the car seat, practice installing it in your car before the baby arrives. Familiarize yourself with its mechanisms. If you are unsure, there are resources online, or you could consider reaching out to a children's hospital. Many have experts who can help ensure you have installed it correctly.

Next on the list is the stroller. With so many types on the market – jogging strollers, umbrella strollers, full travel systems – it can feel overwhelming. Consider your lifestyle when making your selection. If you are a runner, a jogging stroller may be for you. If you travel frequently or live in a city, something lightweight and easily collapsible might be best. Prioritize features like safety harnesses, brakes, and maneuverability when making your selection. Once you have bought it, assemble it and test it out. Try folding and unfolding it, adjusting the seat, and attaching and detaching any extras like a cup holder or a canopy. The more familiar you are with it, the easier it will be to use when the baby arrives.

Let us talk about cribs. This is where your little one will spend a significant portion of their time, so safety is paramount. When choosing a crib, ensure it meets the current safety standards. Slats should be no more than 2 3/8 inches apart to prevent the baby's head from getting stuck. Corner posts should be flush with the end panels, or very tall (such as on a canopy), so the baby's clothing cannot catch. Once it is assembled, check it regularly for loose screws or broken parts. A tip to remember: The mattress should be firm and snugly fit within the crib. You should not be able to fit more than two fingers between the mattress and the crib frame.

When assembling all these items, always follow the manufacturer's instructions. Resist the temptation to wing it. These products are designed with safety in mind, and any modifications or incorrect assembly can compromise that.

Remember, preparing these items is not just about assembly. It is about creating a safe and welcoming space for your baby. It is about envisioning the days ahead when you will buckle your baby into that car seat, take leisurely walks with the stroller, and gently lay your baby down in their crib. Every twist of a screw and every check of a safety strap brings you one step closer to those wonderful moments.

So, take a breath, grab those instruction manuals, and delve into the assembly. Your future self, standing by the car on delivery day with a correctly installed car seat, will thank you. Your baby, secure and snug in their new gear, will thank you too. This is not just preparation. This is the first step in ensuring the safety and comfort of your child, a responsibility that begins now and continues as they grow. You have got this, future dad.

Chapter 10:
Getting Ready for the Ninth Month's Grand Finale

True Signs of Labor Versus False Alarms

As an expectant father, a roller coaster of emotions, an avalanche of thoughts, and a flurry of questions may be running through your mind. And one such critical question is, "How will I know when it is time?" This section is designed to guide you through the crucial signs of labor, helping you distinguish between false alarms and the real deal. It will arm you with the knowledge to act promptly, ensuring the safety and well-being of both your partner and your soon-to-be-born child.

Imagine yourself in the middle of a quiet night, suddenly jolted awake by your partner who says, "I think it is time." Your heart races, a mix of excitement and fear. Is it really time? Are you about to witness the miracle of birth, or is it another practice run? Remember, it is natural to feel a little lost, a little unsure. However, understanding the signs of labor will help you make the right call.

One of the first signs of true labor is consistent contractions. They do not ease up or slow down, rather they become more regular and progressively stronger. To distinguish them from false contractions or "Braxton Hicks," watch out for their frequency and intensity. Braxton Hicks are erratic; they come and go without any consistent pattern and often ease up with a change in activity or position. But real labor contractions are persistent and increase in intensity over time, unaffected by your movement or activity.

Your partner might experience what is known as "water breaking," which is the rupture of the membrane that holds the amniotic fluid. This could be a gush of fluid or a steady trickle. It is a sign that labor is imminent, if not already underway. If the water breaks, contact your healthcare provider immediately, irrespective of the presence of contractions.

Yet another sign is the discharge of the "bloody show" or mucus plug; a jelly-like substance, often streaked with blood. This seals the cervix during pregnancy and its discharge can indicate the onset of labor. But keep in mind, labor may still be a few days away even after the "show."

Most importantly, trust your partner's instincts. If she feels it is time, it is time to act. If contractions are less than 5 minutes apart, lasting for about a minute, and this pattern persists for an hour, it is usually a good indicator of active labor.

When you notice these signs, call your healthcare provider right away. They will guide you on the next steps – whether to rush to the hospital or wait a little longer at home. Remember, every pregnancy is unique. What is important is being alert, patient, and supportive.

Understanding the signs of labor can ease some of the anxieties of childbirth. So, stay prepared, stay informed, and trust in the journey. You are about to embark on the life-changing voyage of fatherhood, so brace yourself, stay calm, and get ready to meet your little one. After all, you have been waiting for this precious moment for nine long months. The finale is around the corner, and you are going to do great. Are you ready to continue to the next section where we delve further into being the pillar of support during labor?

Being Her Pillar of Support Throughout Labor

Imagine, for a moment, that you are standing at the edge of a stormy sea. The waves are crashing, the wind howling, and the skies roaring with thunder. Would you rather face this alone, or would you want someone by your side? Your partner is about to embark on a journey just as tempestuous as this stormy sea – the tumultuous voyage of labor and childbirth. Your presence, your support, can be the anchor that steadies her ship.

Let us talk about emotional support first. Emotional support starts with your understanding and compassion. The process of labor can be overwhelming, with waves of contractions coming and going. Sometimes, it can feel like a wild, untamed river, but remember, she is the one braving the rapids. In these turbulent moments, your empathy is the bridge that connects you two. Be there with her, reassure her, and encourage her. Express your love, admiration, and trust in her strength. Whisper soothing words, cheer her on, and do not forget the power of silence, too. Sometimes, simply holding her hand or offering a comforting touch can say more than a thousand words.

Now, on to physical support. During labor, a woman's body goes through immense stress and strain. And this is where you, as her partner, can make a difference. One of the most effective ways to provide physical support is by aiding with pain management. This can be as simple as helping her change positions, massaging her back or shoulders, or providing counter-pressure during contractions. Remember, these techniques can be learned beforehand from a childbirth class or a doula.

What about the birthing room? In the whirlwind of medical staff, monitoring machines, and possible interventions, it might seem daunting. But think of yourself as the guardian of her birthing space. It is essential to ensure that the room remains a safe and comfortable environment. Dimming the lights, playing her favorite soothing music, using aromatherapy, or even bringing familiar objects from home can help create a calming atmosphere.

One of your crucial roles in the birthing room is to advocate for your partner's wishes. You and your partner would have discussed her birth plan well in advance – her preferences, the desired level of medical intervention, pain management options, and so on. During labor, she might be too focused on the process to voice her wishes. You, as her advocate, can communicate her preferences to the medical team, ensuring her voice is heard and respected.

Remember, however, that birth is a dynamic process and things may not always go as planned. There may be unexpected situations and necessary medical interventions. In such scenarios, your ability to stay calm, understand the situation, and make informed decisions is vital. Trust the medical professionals and ask questions if something is unclear.

Finally, remember this – supporting your partner during labor is not about "saving the day." It is about being there, by her side, as her companion and confidante. It is about sharing the experience, growing together, and bracing yourselves for the miraculous moment that is about to come – the birth of your child.

So, take a deep breath, and dive in. As they say, the smoothest stone is not shaped by still waters but by raging currents. This challenging journey, when navigated together, can lead to the most rewarding destination – parenthood.

Experiencing the Miraculous Moment of Birth

There you are, standing at the edge of the precipice of the most profound moment of your life – the birth of your child. The air in the room is electric with anticipation, thick with a mix of apprehension, excitement, and love. One can never truly prepare for such a transformative moment, but having a better understanding of what to expect and how to navigate this process can be an invaluable aid.

Have you ever watched a sunrise? There is a moment just before dawn when the world is shrouded in dim light. It is as if the earth is holding its breath in anticipation, waiting for that first ray of light to pierce the horizon. That is how the birthing room feels; it is the calm before a beautiful storm of life.

The atmosphere is tense, but it is also wrapped in a sense of wonder, a collective holding of breaths as everyone waits for the star of the show – your baby – to make their grand debut. The tension rises, then falls, like waves against a shore, aligning with the rhythm of your partner's contractions. The closer you get, the sharper each rise, each fall, until suddenly, like the brilliant break of dawn, your child is here.

The intensity of the emotions you will feel might overwhelm you. Fear, anxiety, elation, relief – they all merge into a singular, potent sensation that leaves you breathless. But remember, it is okay to feel scared, to be emotional. It is not a sign of weakness, but rather a testament to the monumental significance of this moment.

One way to mitigate the fear and apprehension is to involve yourself in the process. Being actively involved during the labor can help you feel less like a spectator and more like a participant. Hold your partner's hand, offer words of encouragement, or simply be a comforting presence for her.

There is a moment when the baby's head crowns and the room erupts into a flurry of activity. Amid this orchestrated chaos, your focus narrows down to the two most important people in your life – your partner and your soon-to-be child. The sight might be unnerving, but this is the pivotal moment that the last nine months have been leading up to.

Do not turn away. This is not just about witnessing birth; it is about participating in the miracle of life. Remember, you are not a mere observer but a pillar of strength and support for your partner. This moment is not just about the child being born; it is also about the birth of you as a father.

Once the baby arrives, the wave of emotions can come crashing down. The first cry of your baby will resonate deep within your soul, a primal call that instigates a love so profound it defies articulation. As you hold your baby for the first time, you will experience an overwhelming sense of joy, a realization that life as you knew it has forever changed.

At this moment, pause and remember every sensation – the weight of your baby in your arms, their soft breath against your skin, the pureness in their gaze. These will become your treasures, memories etched in the marrow of your being.

The birthing room is the arena where you will witness the symphony of life unfold in all its raw and unfiltered glory. You will feel fear, yes, but it is this very fear, this feeling of standing on the edge of the unknown, that adds depth to the joy and relief when you finally hold your baby in your arms. So, prepare to embrace it all – the chaos, the emotions, and most importantly, the love.

The journey ahead is long, filled with trials, tribulations, and boundless joy. Welcome to fatherhood. Remember, there is no perfect way to be a father, but millions of ways to be a good one. You have got this.

Providing Postpartum Support Following Birth

Think about that moment when you first held your child in your arms. The elation, the sense of accomplishment, the overwhelming love. Now imagine it through the lens of your partner, who, after the physical ordeal of labor, feels an added layer of exhaustion, both physical and emotional. It is an experience that transcends any she has had before, and she will need your unwavering support to navigate this uncharted territory. This section offers practical advice on how to be that pillar of support she needs in her postpartum recovery.

You may have heard of the term "baby blues," a common phenomenon experienced by new mothers, characterized by mood swings, anxiety, and tearfulness, among other symptoms. This is due to a massive drop in pregnancy hormones coupled with the physical toll of childbirth, sleep deprivation, and the newfound responsibility of caring for a newborn. It is crucial for you to understand these changes and realize that her emotional state may be fragile during this period.

Offer reassurance. Let her know that it is okay to feel overwhelmed and that these feelings are common and temporary. Encourage her to talk about her feelings without fear of judgment. This simple act of validation can be extraordinarily comforting. However, if her feelings of sadness persist beyond the initial couple of weeks or if she exhibits signs of severe depression, consider seeking professional help.

Another practical way of offering support is by assuming more responsibility for baby care tasks and household chores. Share the load of diaper changes, bathing the baby, and nighttime feedings if you can. If the baby is being breastfed, you could bring the baby to your partner and look after burping and settling the baby back to sleep. Managing the household chores would be a massive relief for her, and allow her to rest and recuperate better.

Understanding and addressing her physical recovery is equally important. Encourage her to take it easy and rest as much as possible. Childbirth takes a toll on the body, and it is important to give it time to heal. Encourage a healthy diet and ensure she is well-hydrated, particularly if she is breastfeeding.

Finally, do not forget about the power of small acts of love and care. A warm foot rub, a surprise favorite meal, and taking a moment to sincerely tell her she is doing a fantastic job can boost her spirits enormously. It is all about making her feel cherished and appreciated.

Remember, communication is vital. Do not assume, ask. "How are you feeling?" "What can I do to help you?" "Would you like me to do this …?" are questions that should be frequently on your lips.

Being a new dad can be just as daunting as being a new mom, and it is okay to feel overwhelmed at times. This is a learning curve for both of you, and there will be times when you do not have all the answers, and that is fine. It is the love, care, and effort that counts.

Postpartum support is more than helping out with chores or taking care of the baby. It is about being a solid, empathetic support system for your partner as she navigates the intense journey of becoming a new mother. By being there for her, emotionally and physically, you are not just strengthening your relationship with her, but also establishing a nurturing environment for your newborn. The start of your journey into parenthood may be fraught with challenges, but with understanding, empathy, and cooperation, it can also be an incredibly rewarding experience.

Chapter 11:
Celebrating the Grand Debut

How to Handle the Baby's First Few Days

Congratulations! You have made it through nine months of pregnancy and the excitement of labor. Now, you are home with your little bundle of joy, and life has never been so thrilling and, let us be honest, intimidating. Welcome to fatherhood, the land of the perpetual learning curve. Let us tackle the first few days together, shall we?

First and foremost, let us talk about feeding. If your partner is breastfeeding, she will be on the front lines of this endeavor, but that does not mean you are a bench player. In fact, you have a key role in the feeding process. You can help ensure mom is hydrated and well-fed to maintain her strength. Bring her a glass of water or a healthy snack during feeding sessions. And yes, even at 2 AM. She will appreciate it more than you will ever know.

If your baby is bottle-fed, whether with formula or expressed breast milk, you get to share more directly in the feeding responsibilities. Use this time to bond with your baby, holding them close, making eye contact, and talking or singing softly. Remember, babies have tiny stomachs, so they need to eat often. Do not worry about the clock; watch your baby. Hunger cues might include more alertness, increased mouthing, or becoming more active.

Next, diaper changing. A messy business, yes, but essential. You will likely be changing diapers around ten times a day. The first few might be a little awkward, but you will get the hang of it, trust me. Always remember to wipe from front to back, especially with girls. Be sure to have everything you need within arm's reach before you start. Do not forget the golden rule: Never leave your baby unattended on the changing table.

Finally, how to tell if your baby is sick. Newborns cannot tell us when something is wrong, so we have to be excellent observers. Things to look out for are changes in behavior or eating habits, fever, unusual fussiness, or trouble breathing. Also, note any changes in their skin color, poop, or pee.

Trust your instincts. You are getting to know your baby, and you will begin to sense when something is not right. If something worries you, never hesitate to reach out to your pediatrician. That is what they are there for.

Remember, no one expects you to be an expert right away. You will fumble, maybe even drop a diaper or two (hopefully not the loaded ones), and that is perfectly okay. Fatherhood is a journey, not a destination. These first few days will be a whirlwind of emotions and new experiences. Take them in stride, know that you are not alone, and enjoy these moments. This is just the beginning of a beautiful adventure.

Your love, patience, and willingness to jump right into the trenches are the most important elements in this equation. So arm yourself with a good sense of humor and a strong cup of coffee. These first few days will pass quickly, but they will leave you with memories that last a lifetime. And remember, you have got this!

Sharing the Joy and Challenges That Come With Parenting

Picture this scenario: It is 2 AM, and your precious newborn is crying out for attention yet again. You have had only a smattering of sleep and you are so tired that your vision blurs. Do you do it alone and let your partner sleep, or do you gently nudge her awake and share the duty? This is one of many scenarios that will test your resolve as co-parents, and the decisions you make can set the tone for your relationship moving forward.

Co-parenting in the initial days of your baby's life is like learning a new dance. There is a rhythm to it, a balance that needs to be struck, and above all, there is teamwork. No single partner can (or should) take on the full weight of the responsibilities. While your partner is recovering from childbirth and dealing with hormonal changes, you will likely find yourself shouldering a larger share of the duties. This might mean changing diapers, making bottles, or just rocking the baby to sleep at odd hours.

So, how do you navigate this shared journey of parenting without stepping on each other's toes? Here are some practical strategies:

Firstly, have open, honest conversations about how you envision the division of responsibilities. It is essential to have these discussions during the day when you are both alert and can talk calmly. Agree on who does what, and be willing to adjust as you go along. Remember, you are a team, and negotiation is key.

Secondly, communicate regularly and openly about how you are feeling. It is okay to admit that you are exhausted, or that you are unsure about how to comfort a crying baby. It is equally okay to express a need for help, a break, or a pat on the back for a job well done. Your feelings are important, and so are your partner's feelings.

Thirdly, do not keep score. Parenting is not a competition. Some days, you will take on more of the load; other days, your partner will. What matters is that you both understand and appreciate each other's efforts. Remember, mutual support and acknowledgment can go a long way in strengthening your bond as co-parents.

And lastly, create opportunities for joint interaction with the baby. Bathing, feeding, or just cuddling your baby together can be wonderful bonding experiences that also share the responsibility.

Let us remember, the concept of shared parenting extends beyond the realm of tasks. It is about more than just "doing" – it is also about "being." It involves being there for each other emotionally, offering words of encouragement, and sharing the joys and challenges that come with parenting.

Remember that viral image of a dad lying down next to his partner who is feeding the baby in the middle of the night, just so she does not feel alone? That is shared parenting. It is a silent, mutual understanding that you are in this together. It is the recognition that every little action, every small sacrifice contributes to the immense task of raising your little one.

In this dance of shared parenting, you will undoubtedly stumble and miss a few steps, and that is okay. This dance is not about perfection, it is about connection and teamwork. Embrace the experience, learn from each other, and remember to enjoy the music. After all, this is a dance you will remember for the rest of your lives.

Learning Your Newborn's Secret Language

Have you ever noticed how each baby's cry has its own unique sound? Even as a new father, it might seem like a symphony of high-pitched wails, but each of those unique sounds conveys a specific message. In this section, we are going to unveil the secret language of babies and help you to decode those cues.

Each baby is different, but there are common signs that you can look for. It is your role to play detective and figure out what your little one is trying to tell you. Do not worry; this is not as hard as it sounds.

Let us start with hunger cues. Picture this: Your baby is turning his head toward your hand as you caress his cheek. You may see him opening and closing his mouth or sucking on his fingers. This behavior, known as "rooting," is a strong indicator that your baby is ready for feeding. Respond to this cue promptly; waiting until the baby cries out of hunger can make feeding more stressful for both of you.

But what about when the baby cries? A hunger cry tends to be a rhythmic, repetitive cry, starting low and increasing in intensity. Think of it as an insistent, "Feed me now." You will soon begin to recognize this sound. And remember, crying is a late sign of hunger, so try to initiate feeding at the first sign of fussiness.

Now, consider sleep cues. You are probably dreaming about the day when your baby will sleep through the night, right? However, newborns have irregular sleep cycles, which is entirely normal. Look out for signs of sleepiness in your baby – yawning, rubbing eyes, or getting fussy. Respond to these cues promptly by beginning the bedtime routine. If you wait until the baby is overtired, they may find it harder to settle down.

While you may become quite adept at decoding these common cues, there will be times when your baby cries, and you are not sure why. The nappy is dry, the baby is not hungry, and sleep is not the issue. Then what? This is where your patience and detective skills come into play. Sometimes, your baby might just need a change of scenery, a gentle rocking, or a calming lullaby.

Remember, it is okay not to have all the answers right away. Parenting is a journey of learning and discovery. You and your partner are figuring things out together. There is no manual to this, and it is perfectly fine to make mistakes. The most important thing is that you are trying your best and that you are there for your little one, offering comfort and reassurance.

Here are a few quick tips:

- Keep track of your baby's feeding and sleeping patterns. Over time, you will start to see patterns and can anticipate your baby's needs better.
- Respond promptly to hunger and sleep cues. This can help establish a healthy routine and reduce stress for both you and your baby.
- If you cannot figure out why your baby is upset, try different soothing techniques. Some babies love being swaddled, while others respond well to gentle rocking or white noise.
- Remember that it is okay to ask for help. If you are feeling overwhelmed, talk to your partner, family, or healthcare professional.

Through patience and love, you will grow more in tune with your baby's cues and needs. This connection is invaluable, building a bond that will continue to deepen over the years.

Fostering Unconditional Love Through Baby Bonding

If you were to ask any seasoned father what the most magical part of their journey was, chances are, they will tell you it was the bonding moments with their newborn. Nothing else, no amount of money, no promotion, no victory, equals the profound joy and profound connection that occurs when you interact and bond with your baby. The soft glow in their eyes, the contagious joy of their laughter, the touch of their tiny fingers – these are the irreplaceable treasures that enrich your journey into fatherhood.

Bonding is not a one-time event but a continuous process that unfolds over time, like a carefully nurtured plant growing stronger day by day. It is the heartfelt connection that you develop with your baby, that not only fulfills their emotional needs but also sets the groundwork for their future social and emotional development.

To begin with, skin-to-skin contact, also known as kangaroo care, is a tried-and-true method of establishing this bond. This is where you hold your naked baby against your own bare skin, often covered by a blanket. Close physical contact has numerous benefits. It comforts your baby, helps regulate their heart rate and breathing, promotes better sleep, and fosters breastfeeding. More than anything, it makes your baby feel secure in the new world they have entered. Make it a routine to spend some time each day holding your baby this way. Perhaps you can do it while your partner takes a much-needed break or after you come home from work. You will be amazed at the peace and connection it can cultivate.

Next, your voice is another powerful tool in the bonding process. Do you remember speaking to the belly of your partner during pregnancy? Well, now it is time to continue those conversations directly. Even though your newborn might not understand the words, they recognize your voice. The sound that was their constant companion in the womb still has the power to soothe and comfort them. Read to your baby, sing lullabies, or simply tell them about your day. The point is to make your voice a familiar, reassuring presence in their life.

Incorporating bonding moments into daily care routines is also an excellent strategy. Bathing, feeding, and diaper changing are all prime opportunities for interaction. Look into your baby's eyes, talk to them, make funny faces, or sing songs. Such moments of joy and laughter become the highlight of their day, as well as yours. They also transform routine care from a task into a rewarding experience.

One final piece of advice – be patient. Bonding is not a race. It takes time. You might not feel an intense connection immediately, and that is perfectly fine. Every father uniquely experiences this journey. Do not judge yourself by others' experiences. Keep providing loving care and interaction, and the bond will grow.

In this journey, remember, you are not just providing care; you are creating memories, teaching life lessons, and above all, building a loving relationship that will stand the test of time. The more you bond with your baby, the more you solidify your role as their safe haven, their guide, their most trusted companion – their father. And that is the most beautiful reward of fatherhood, right?

Chapter 12:
Setting Sail on the Continued Journey of Fatherhood

Baby Sleep Schedules – How to Get Through Sleepless Nights

At 3 AM, you awaken to the sounds of your newborn's crying. Your mind is foggy, and your body is heavy, yearning for more sleep. But this is your new reality. You are a parent now, and this is just another facet of fatherhood, one where the night becomes your friend, and the patter of small feet fills your dreams. Let us talk about surviving sleepless nights and managing your baby's sleep schedules.

First and foremost, remember, you are not alone in this. Every parent, at some point, has stood exactly where you are standing now. Bleary-eyed and sleep-deprived, yet filled with an unquenchable love for this tiny person. Embrace this time, difficult though it may be, because, believe it or not, it passes all too quickly.

Now, let us get practical. Babies, especially newborns, do not have set sleeping patterns. Their tiny tummies need frequent feeding, leading to a sleep-feed-wake cycle that runs around the clock. But there are a few strategies you can employ to make things more manageable.

Begin by understanding your baby's sleep patterns. Newborns sleep a lot, up to 16 to 17 hours a day. However, their sleep cycle is divided into many short periods. In the first few weeks, expect your baby to wake up every 2 to 3 hours for feeding. As they grow, their sleep will consolidate into longer periods, eventually settling into a more routine sleep schedule.

Next, aim to establish a regular bedtime routine. Consistency is key here. You could start with a gentle bath, followed by a feeding session, a lullaby or story, and then bed. This routine can signal your baby that it is time to wind down and sleep. While this may not work immediately, with time, your baby will start to understand the cues.

Sharing night duties is another effective way to cope with sleepless nights. Work out a schedule with your partner so that both of you can get some uninterrupted sleep. Perhaps one of you can take the first half of the night, and the other can take the second half. Or one can be in charge of feeding, and the other can handle diaper changes. If breastfeeding, the mother can pump breast milk for the father to feed the baby at night, offering her a chance to rest.

Embrace the power of naps. Sleep when your baby sleeps, they say. It may sound cliché, but it is excellent advice. Short naps during the day can help combat fatigue and give you the energy you need to take care of your baby and yourself.

Finally, remember that it is okay to ask for help. If a friend or family member offers to watch your baby for a couple of hours so you can rest, say "Yes." If sleep deprivation becomes too much to handle, consult a healthcare professional or a sleep coach. There is no shame in seeking assistance; it does not make you any less of a parent.

Sleepless nights with a newborn can be challenging, but these are moments of bonding, of quiet love. These experiences, even the difficult ones, shape you as a father. Every night you rise to comfort your baby, you grow stronger, more patient, more compassionate. And while the nights may be long, they are not forever. So, take heart, dear reader. You are doing a great job. Now, breathe in, brave the night, and know that with each sunrise, you are one day closer to a full night's sleep.

Help Her Get Over the Baby Blues

You have navigated sleepless nights together, and now another challenge beckons. You will soon learn that the journey to fatherhood does not stop with the birth of your child. You will also realize that there are changes in your partner that you will have to understand and navigate, just as much as she does. She may be experiencing postpartum emotional changes, including "baby blues" or even postpartum depression. This is a delicate period that will test both your strength and empathy. So how do you provide emotional support, encourage professional help when necessary, and remain understanding during this time?

Let us begin by understanding what the "baby blues" are. This term refers to a mild, temporary mood disorder experienced by up to 80% of new mothers. Symptoms may include mood swings, anxiety, sadness, irritability, feeling overwhelmed, crying, reduced concentration, appetite problems, and trouble sleeping. These feelings often begin within the first two to three days after delivery and may last for up to two weeks.

Now, while "baby blues" are relatively common and manageable, postpartum depression (PPD) is a more severe, long-lasting form of depression. PPD is not a character or parenting flaw; it is a complication of giving birth. Symptoms can include severe mood swings, difficulty bonding with the baby, withdrawal from family and friends, loss of appetite, severe anxiety and panic attacks, thoughts of harming oneself or the baby, and recurrent thoughts of death or suicide.

Now that you understand the difference, it is crucial to offer emotional support to your partner. Listen to her, validate her feelings, and assure her it is okay to feel this way. She is not alone, and neither are you. Many new parents feel overwhelmed and anxious; it is a natural part of this life-changing experience. Reassure her that it is okay to take time for self-care and that her well-being matters.

However, if your partner is showing signs of postpartum depression, it is vital to encourage professional help. While it might be difficult, it is essential to speak up. Openly communicate your concerns and encourage her to seek help from a healthcare provider. This step is crucial as PPD requires professional treatment, which may include psychotherapy, medication, or both. Remember that seeking help is not a sign of weakness but of strength and an act of love for both your partner and the baby.

Being understanding and patient during this time is paramount. This is a significant adjustment period for her, and she is not her symptoms. It is important to remember this is a temporary phase, and with the right help and support, she will overcome it.

If you are feeling overwhelmed, remember, it is okay to seek support for yourself, too. It is a lot to take on, and it is essential to maintain your mental well-being as well. Speak with friends, family, or a mental health professional about your feelings.

Remember, empathy, patience, and love are your guiding principles during this period. The path may be challenging, but you are not walking it alone. Reach out to those around you, communicate openly, and most importantly, remember that this, too, will pass.

Cultivating Your Relationship While Embracing Parenthood

Picture this: It is the end of a long day. The baby's finally asleep, the house is quiet, and you and your partner are in the living room, exhausted. Now, this could be the time when you both crash on the couch, with a show running on the TV as background noise. Or it could be a moment of connection, of nurturing the bond that brought you on this journey of parenthood.

Stepping into the realm of parenthood is a beautiful voyage, a roller coaster filled with the joys of first smiles, coos, and baby milestones. But with the journey comes a whirlwind of emotions and tasks that can sometimes push your romantic relationship into the backdrop. This does not mean the love fades, but rather it becomes obscured by the fog of sleepless nights and diaper changes.

So, how do you maintain your relationship amid the storm of new parenthood? First and foremost, communication is key. Parenthood introduces a new dynamic to your relationship, and open dialogue about these changes can help mitigate misunderstandings and frustrations. Discuss your roles and expectations, voice concerns, and validate each other's feelings. You are a team, navigating through this novel territory together, and no concern is too trivial to share.

Secondly, sharing responsibilities is crucial. Caring for a newborn is rewarding but also demanding. Instead of splitting duties strictly down the middle, play to your strengths. Maybe one of you is a whiz at calming the baby while the other excels at meal preparation. Remember, it is not a competition. The goal is to create a harmonious environment where both of you feel valued and supported.

Yet, amid the hustle of parenthood, do not forget the spark that brought you together in the first place. Yes, you are parents, but you are also partners. Sustaining the romance does not necessitate grand gestures. A simple compliment, a shared joke, or a quick hug can remind you both of the bond you share. When time and energy permit, have a date night. It could be as extravagant as a night out or as simple as a quiet dinner at home after the baby is asleep.

New parenthood also presents an opportunity to deepen your relationship. Yes, there will be disagreements and tense moments, but navigating through them together can strengthen your bond. In such moments, try to remind each other of the love you share, and the beautiful journey you have embarked on together.

Embrace the change, adapt, and grow together. Keep the lines of communication open, share responsibilities, and remember to nourish the love that brought you here. Understand that the dynamics of your relationship will evolve, and that is okay. You are not just partners anymore; you are parents, a family.

And one day, when you are both sitting in the quiet living room, looking at the peaceful face of your sleeping baby, you will realize that despite the challenges, you would not change a thing. For your love has not diminished, but grown, encompassing a tiny new life that has made your journey even more meaningful.

Contemplating the Journey and the Evolution Into Fatherhood

It seems just like yesterday when you received the news of impending fatherhood. The excitement, the nervous anticipation, the torrent of emotions – remember those days? Those were the first steps on a transformative journey, one that has led you to this moment, cradling your newborn child in your arms and feeling a rush of indescribable love. You have navigated the tumultuous seas of pregnancy, braved the storms of late nights, diaper changes, and bouts of crying, and emerged a stronger, more resilient individual. You have changed, grown, and become a father.

Look at the mirror now. You may notice the slight graying of your hair, perhaps a few more lines on your face. They are not merely signs of aging; they are badges of honor, physical tokens of the love, care, and patience you have poured into your journey as a father. The transformation is not just physical, though. Inside, you have also matured, emotionally and psychologically. Each trial you faced, each challenge you overcame, chiseled away the rough edges, refining your character, molding you into a more empathetic, more patient, more understanding person. You have learned to listen more, to empathize more, to love more profoundly.

Remember those moments of despair when the baby would not stop crying, or when your partner was overwhelmed with postpartum blues? Think about the strength you found within yourself during those times, the resilience you discovered. Those moments might have been challenging, but they were also moments of growth, moments that tested and eventually proved your mettle as a father.

And then there are the rewards, the precious moments that make every hardship worth it. The first time your baby gripped your finger, the first time they looked into your eyes, the first time they smiled at you – each of these milestones holds a special place in your heart. They serve as beautiful reminders of why you embarked on this journey in the first place.

Reflect on this journey you have been on, the road you have traveled from being an expectant father to becoming a parent. You have come a long way. But remember, this is only the beginning. Fatherhood is a journey, not a destination. Each day will present new challenges, new learning experiences, new opportunities to grow, and more heartwarming moments to cherish.

As you step forward into this next chapter of your life, carry with you the lessons you have learned so far. Remain patient, stay strong, keep learning, and remember to cherish every moment. Being a father is not about perfection; it is about love, care, understanding, and the ability to stand up each time you fall.

And finally, look forward to the future. Imagine your child's first steps, their first words, their first day at school. All these future milestones are waiting for you, waiting to fill your life with more joy, more love, and more precious memories.

In closing, remember that you are not alone on this journey. The road of fatherhood is well-trodden, with many who have walked it before and many who will walk it after. Draw strength from this brotherhood of fathers, and when the time comes, pass on your wisdom to those who will follow. As a father, you are now part of a timeless continuum, a legacy of love that stretches back through the ages and will extend into the future. Embrace this role and embark on this continuous journey with confidence, joy, and anticipation. Congratulations, and welcome to fatherhood.

Embarking on a Parenthood Journey Together

Dear reader,

As we reach the final pages of this guide, I sincerely hope it has provided you with valuable insights, encouragement, and useful strategies as you prepare to embark on this incredible journey of parenthood.

Just as you are gearing up to support your partner and welcome your new baby, I would love for you to support others on their similar journey by sharing your honest impressions about this book on Amazon. Your feedback not only assists other first-time dads in their quest for knowledge but also contributes significantly to the success of this book.

Leaving a review will require only a few moments of your time, but it can have a profound impact on future readers searching for a comprehensive guide. As a self-published author, I promise to read your review personally, and I greatly appreciate all forms of feedback, be it positive or constructive.

Thank you for your valuable time and for allowing this book to be a part of your life-changing journey. I eagerly await your thoughts and opinions.

Scan to leave a review !

Best wishes,

Peter Neel

Final Words

As we draw the final curtain on this guide, I want to honor the immense journey you are about to embark upon. Fatherhood, a voyage filled with joy, wonder, trials, and triumphs, is a path that will indelibly shape your life.

Throughout this book, we have explored a multitude of ways to navigate the complex journey of pregnancy and to provide unparalleled support to your partner. We have ventured into the realm of understanding and empathizing with the physical and emotional changes that pregnancy brings, and we have shared strategies to foster a nurturing and secure environment for the arrival of your baby.

Now comes the time to implement the knowledge and strategies you have learned. I urge you to take these lessons to heart, utilize these tools, and venture into fatherhood with confidence and compassion. It is time to embrace your new role, treasure every moment of your partner's pregnancy, and celebrate the miracle of life that is soon to be yours.

Being a supportive partner during pregnancy is the first stepping stone in your journey to becoming an extraordinary father. Remember, fatherhood is not a role that one perfects overnight. It is a lifelong commitment, an ongoing learning experience filled with endless love, understanding, and patience.

And so, as we part ways, I leave you with a heartfelt wish. May the knowledge and wisdom shared in this book guide you in the magical journey of fatherhood. May you find strength, joy, and fulfillment in your role as a first-time dad.

Good luck on this extraordinary adventure. Cherish the moments, embrace the challenges, and above all, celebrate the beautiful journey of becoming a father. The world awaits your greatness, and your child awaits your love.

It is not just about being a man; it is about being the best man you can be for your child. Now, go forth and embrace your destiny. The realm of fatherhood awaits.

About the Author

Peter Neel is a dedicated writer and father whose journey through parenthood has shaped much of his work. Born and raised in Seattle, Washington, his rich background in journalism and storytelling has been colored by his experiences as a parent, lending his narratives a deep-seated authenticity.

In his works, Neel explores the diverse terrain of fatherhood, reflecting on the laughter, tears, surprises, and everyday miracles that make up this unique adventure. He is known for his ability to articulate complex emotions and scenarios with humor and sensitivity, providing comfort and camaraderie to fellow parents through his words.

Neel's own path to fatherhood was marked by the excitement and uncertainties that every new parent encounters. The life-altering experience of becoming a dad not only revolutionized his personal world but also had a profound impact on his writing. His stories often depict the intricate relationships between parents and their children, resonating deeply with readers who see their own experiences reflected in his honest and heartwarming tales.

Despite his successful writing career, Neel places his role as a father at the center of his identity. His writing breaks frequently for family movie nights, pancake breakfasts, and coaching his kids' soccer games. These moments of ordinary magic provide endless inspiration for his work, offering unique insights into the trials and triumphs of parenthood.

In his free time, Neel often takes his family on travel adventures, exploring different cultures and landscapes. These trips provide further enriching experiences that influence his understanding of familial bonds and personal growth.

Peter Neel is not only an author but also a mentor to fellow fathers navigating the often-untrodden paths of parenthood. His work embodies the joy, challenges, and profound love inherent in the journey of fatherhood, making him a relatable and revered voice in contemporary literature.

Printed in Great Britain
by Amazon